Surgical
Oral Pathology

Surgical Oral Pathology

KMK Masthan
Professor and Head

N Aravindha Babu
Professor

L Malathi
Senior Lecturer

E Rajesh
Senior Lecturer

Department of Oral Pathology
Sree Balaji Dental College and Hospital
Bharath University, Pallikaranai, Chennai

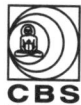

CBS Publishers & Distributors Pvt Ltd

New Delhi • Bengaluru • Chennai • Kochi • Kolkata • Mumbai
Hyderabad • Nagpur • Patna • Pune • Vijayawada

Surgical Oral Pathology

ISBN: 978-81-239-2934-7

First Edition: 2016

Published by Satish Kumar Jain and produced by Varun Jain for

CBS Publishers & Distributors Pvt Ltd
4819/XI Prahlad Street, 24 Ansari Road, Daryaganj, New Delhi 110 002, India.
Ph: 23289259, 23266861, 23266867 Website: www.cbspd.com
Fax: 011-23243014   e-mail: delhi@cbspd.com; cbspubs@airtelmail.in.
Corporate Office: 204 FIE, Industrial Area, Patparganj, Delhi 110 092
Ph: 4934 4934   Fax: 4934 4935   e-mail: publishing@cbspd.com; publicity@cbspd.com

Branches

- **Bengaluru:** Seema House 2975, 17th Cross, KR Road,
  Banasankari 2nd Stage, Bengaluru 560 070, Karnataka
  Ph: +91-80-26771678/79   Fax: +91-80-26771680   e-mail: bangalore@cbspd.com
- **Chennai:** 7, Subbaraya Street, Shenoy Nagar, Chennai 600 030, Tamil Nadu
  Ph: +91-44-26680620, 26681266   Fax: +91-44-42032115   e-mail: chennai@cbspd.com
- **Kochi:** Ashana House, No. 39/1904, AM Thomas Road, Valanjambalam,
  Eranakulam 682 018, Kochi, Kerala
  Ph: +91-484-4059061-65, 67   Fax: +91-484-4059065   e-mail: kochi@cbspd.com
- **Kolkata:** 6/B, Ground Floor, Rameswar Shaw Road, Kolkata 700 014, West Bengal
  Ph: +91-33-22891126, 22891127, 22891128   e-mail: kolkata@cbspd.com
- **Mumbai:** 83-C, Dr E Moses Road, Worli, Mumbai 400018, Maharashtra
  Ph: +91-22-24902340/41   Fax: +91-22-24902342   e-mail: mumbai@cbspd.com

Representatives

- **Hyderabad** 0-9885175004 • **Nagpur**   0-9021734563 • **Patna**   0-9334159340
- **Pune**   0-9623451994 • **Vijayawada** 0-9000660880

Printed at: India Binding House, Noida

to
Dr S Jagathrakshakan
Chancellor, Bharath
University
whose unfailing faith and
continuous encouragement is
the motivation for this book

Foreword

It is a pleasure and an honour to write the foreword to *Surgical Oral Pathology*. This book throws light on what a surgeon must keep in his mind while planning the management of oral pathological lesions. Such well-informed approach towards surgical plan will play a major role in the prognosis, remission and cure.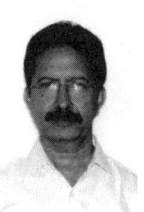

This book has been compiled with great accuracy and efficacy so as not to leave out minute details. I am sure that this book will be of great use to the medical and dental students, clinicians, dentists in everyday practice. This book would prove to be a valuable addition to the medical and dental scientific literatures and I wish the team who worked for bringing out this book with great success in the forthcoming medical literary endeavours.

Kanagasabai V
MD, MBA (Hosp Admn)
Registrar
Bharath University
(Bharath Institute of Higher Education and Research)

Preface

Surgical pathology is that aspect of pathology the surgeon has to bear in his mind while planning surgical treatments. In addition, thorough understanding of the lesion being operated will help the surgeon to discuss with the patient the probable outcome of the surgery, like feasibility of recurrence, likelihood of spread to distant organs and the sequel on the system due to the lesion and the surgery, etc. Reciprocally the pathologist, by being aware of this aspect of pathology, can give more focused diagnosis. Most instances, when a pathologist reports a biopsy, he pursues the popular trend of giving an academically appealing diagnosis. But such diagnosis has no value to the surgeon to make an informed treatment approach. The surgeon invariably feels that, while being confronted with bombastic terminologies of the biopsy report, his clinical decision would be better and result oriented. This creates a gulf between available knowledge and actual treatment being carried out. The focus of this book is to bridge that gap and make available the knowledge resources of the pathologist to the surgeon to enhance his decision making and produce better result outcomes from his/her surgeries. The ultimate aim of both the surgeon and the pathologist is to serve the patient better and produce more cures, which is the goal of this book.

When confronted by dubious lesions with confusing clinical, morphological and conflicting history from the patient, the surgeon actually hopes and looks forward to a helpful suggestion from the pathologist. Unmindful of such expectancy and need, an academic, namesake report will disappoint the surgeon and may actually irritate him since he has lost valuable time waiting for the pathology report. That should never be the case and the pathologist must convey whatever he considers would be the appropriate approach the surgeon must pursue. That is the primary motive behind writing this book. After all, irrespective of the specialities we have one master to serve and that is the welfare of the patient.

The removal of diagnostic site of lesion tissue during biopsy by the surgeon is vital to obtain correct diagnosis from the pathologist. A biopsy from non-representative areas may lead to innocuous reports by the pathologist, which is a precious waste of time and resources of both the surgeon and the pathologist. Differentiating the lesion and normal tissue and thereby giving proper marginal clearance in surgery is also very important to avoid recurrences.

The context of this book is oral pathological lesions that would go under the knife of a surgeon. The burn, i.e. radiotherapy and the poison, i.e. the chemotherapy in case of oral malignancies have also been widely discussed in suitable lesions. Since oral lesions can have a diverse morphology both from the viewpoint of histopathology and distribution wise, this challenging task of discussing them has been done to the best of our knowledge and ability. However, since this surgical oral pathology subject is a maiden by precedence and since this book is a pioneer effort in this discipline, there may be lapses and inadvertent mistakes. Readers may feel free to point out them at masthankmk@gmail.com.

I am greatly indebted to Dr N Anitha, senior lecturer of oral pathology and microbiology, for her help in compiling the data.

My wholehearted thanks to CBS Publishers & Distributors, the doyen in the field of medical publications, for taking up our work for publication.

KMK Masthan

Contents

1

Introduction

HISTORY BEHIND

In the 1870's, Carl Ruge and his associates in the university of Berlin, introduced the surgical biopsy as an essential diagnostic tool. In 1889 on the need of establish a microscopic diagnosis before operating in suspected cases of malignant tumors requiring extensive mutilating procedures. Shortly thereafter, the freezing microtome was introduced and the frozen section procedures hastened the acceptance of this recommendation.

William S Halsted was the first American surgeon to create a division of surgical pathology, this pioneer efforts, which were initially met with indifference and occasionally scorn by the academic pathology establishment, proved to be hugely successful.

Many individuals who contributed to consolidate the speciality of surgical pathology in the United States during the first half of the century.

Pathologist Role in Surgical Pathology

The basic characteristic of the surgical pathologist were masterfully described by the doctor Lauren V. Ackerman the surgical pathologist has the unique opportunity of bridging the gap between the beginning of disease and its end stages, and he should take advantage of this circumstance. It can be done this only after a solid foundation of study at the autopsy table, where the ravages of cancer and other disease are all too clear. With this background pathologist correlate the initial stages of the disease seen in specimens from living patients in the surgical pathology laboratory and make fundamental contribution to knowledge.

Surgical Pathology Report

The delivery of the specimen in the surgical pathology laboratory initiates the complex series of events that culminates in the issuance of the final report. The surgical pathology report is an important medical document that should describe, as thoroughly and concisely as possible, all the relevant gross and microscopic features of a case but should also interpret the significance for the clinician. It should be prompt, accurate, and brief. The pathologist should avoid unnecessary histologic jargon that is of no consequence to the case and concentrate on the aspects that bear a relation to therapy and prognosis.

The usual surgical pathology report is composed of five major fields. The first, designated as "history", contains the essential clinical data known to the pathologist at the time he dictates a description of the gross specimen such as sex and age of the patient, symptoms, surgical findings, and the type of surgery. It should also list previous biopsies on the same patients, if any had been taken.

The second field, designated as "gross", contains the gross description of the specimen. This should be precise and thorough, because once the gross specimen is discarded, this description remains the only document by which the gross features of the case can be evaluated. It should indicate how the various specimens were identified by these surgeon and whether they were received fresh or fixed, intact or open. The specimen should be described in a logical sequential fashion, with a clear description of gross abnormalities and their location. The size, color, and location of all lesion should be recorded. The metric system is to be used for all measurements. It is advisable to give specific dimension and description and weight of the whole specimen should be recorded.

The third field is termed "microscopic", it is regarded as the optional feature of the report, that in many case is unnecessary. When included, it should be short and to the point.

The fourth and the most important field of the report is the "diagnosis", each specimen received should have a separate diagnosis or diagnoses. Our practice is to divide each diagnosis into two parts, separated by a dash. The first, lists the organ, specific site in that organ, and operation, the second gives the morphologic diagnosis. This provide the reader with all essential information on that particular specimen in a single entry.

The fifth field, applicable to only some cases, is a "note" or "comment". In it, the pathologist name mentioned the differential diagnosis, give the reasons for the diagnostic interpretation, make some prognostic and therapeutic considerations about the entity, and include selected references.

If a frozen section has been performed in the information regarding the organ biopsied, the diagnosis given, the names of pathologist who performed the procedure, and the final diagnosis corresponding to the frozen sample should be included in the report, either as a separate field or incorporated into the history of gross field.

It is medically and legally important that the diagnosis and comments made by the pathologist on a given case should be documented as clearly as possible in a written form in the clinical chart via the pathology report. This should be done because some times there is a remarkable discrepancy between the diagnostic consideration given verbally by the pathologist to the clinician and the paraphrasing of these consideration by the clinician in the chart. When an urgent decision needs to be made on the basis of a pathologic finding, the clinician should not have to wait for that information to reach him by routine typewritten report. In that case surgical pathology reports can be distributed by computed-driven telephone fax device. However, it is well to remember that no technologic advancement can replace the time-honoured practice of two medical specialists discussing, immediately after the facts are known, how to best treat a patient.

Slide Review and Consultation

A very fortunate aspect of pathology is the fact that the material on which the diagnosis is made by microscopic slide of a permanent nature and can be evaluated by different observers or by a same observer at different times. All slides and paraffin wax should be stored indefinitely. Whenever a specimen is received in the laboratory, the files should be searched for previous materials on the same patient. If such materials are present, the slides and report should be reviewed. It is mandatory also to the pathologist to review the outside slides of patient who is referred to the institution with the microscopic diagnosis made elsewhere before therapy is begun. It is the responsibility of the pathology department of the referring institution—as legal custodians of this material—to carefully packed and shift this material with the copy of their pathology report.

Limitations of Histological Diagnosis

It is important for the surgical pathologist to know the limitations of his speciality as it is for him to be aware of its strength and potential contributions. This fact has been expressed in a most perceptive and amusing way by Dr Oscar N Rambo. Pathologist are physicians and human beings, they have as great a capacity for error and susceptibility to subjective distractions as other practitioners of the art of medicine. Incomplete communication between the clinician and the pathologist may make diagnosis difficult or impossible. Most physicians are thought that the best biopsy is a cleanly excised, uncrushed wedge that includes the junction between normal and neoplastic tissue.

Biopsy

Interpreting biopsies is one of the most important duties of the surgical pathologist. In incisional biopsies, only a portion of lesion is sampled, and therefore the procedure is strictly of a diagnostic nature. In excisional biopsies, the entire lesion is removed, usually with a rim of normal tissue, and therefore the procedure serves both a diagnostic and therapeutic functions.

Biopsies are also classified according to the instrument used to obtain them; cold knife, cautery, needle or endoscope. Of these, the one usually least suitable for microscopic interpretation is that obtained with a cautery, because this instrument chars and distorts the tissue and prevents the proper staining.

General Rules for Biopsy Procedures

- The larger the lesion, the more numerous biopsies that should be taken from it because of the variability in pattern that may exist and the fact that the diagnostic areas may be present focally.
- In an ulcerated tumors, biopsy of the central ulcerated area may show only necrosis and inflammation. The most informative biopsy is likely to be one taken from the periphery that includes both normal and diseased tissue.
- The biopsy should be deep enough that the relationship between tumor and stroma can be properly assessed.
- Deeply seated lesions are sometimes accompanied by a prominent peripheral tissue reaction, which may be characterized by chronic inflammation, hyperemia, fibrosis, calcification and

metaplastic bone formation. Deep seated lymph node may show involvement by a malignant tumor, whereas a superficial node may show only nonspecific hyperplasia.

- When several fragments of tissues are obtained, they should all send to pathology department and submitted for microscopical examination. Sometime the smaller or grossly less impressive fragment is the only one that contains the diagnostic elements.
- Crushing or squeezing of the tissue with the forceps at time of biopsy by the surgeon or gross examination by the pathologist or at the time of embedding by the histotechnologist should be carefully avoided. The artefact resulting from it often render a biopsy impossible to interpret.
- Biopsy should be placed immediately into a container with an adequate volume of fixative. If not, it would not provide any information about diagnosis but will create artefact.
- Depending on the presumed or known nature of the lesion, consideration should be given to the possible need for special studies, such as touch preparations, electron microscopy, cytogenetics, molecular pathology, flow cytometry.

Quality Control

The monitoring of the quality of the work being carried out in a laboratory of surgical pathology for the purposes of detecting inadequacy, updating procedures and improving the final product, is an important responsibility of the laboratory director or its delicate. Traditionally, this has been carried out in an informal and highly personalised fashion. It is mandated a more structured and rigorous system of self checking, under designations such as quality control, quality assurance, quality improvement and total quality assessment.

Legal Aspects in Surgical Pathology

The most common reasons for surgical pathologist being brought to a trial of the clients that 1. A mistaken diagnosis was made on the basis of misinterpretation of the slide; 2. important lesion or feature present in the specimen was missed, either because of oversight or through failure of sampling; and 3. The pathological diagnosis failed to give the clinician a clear idea about the nature or extent of the lesion or the adequacy of the sample because of poor wording or omission in the report.

2
Gross Techniques in Surgical Pathology

INTRODUCTION

The routine work associated with a surgical pathology specimen includes gross and microscopic examination. The smaller the specimen, the less significant the gross examination appears to be. It has been stated that autopsy pathology is gross pathology, whereas surgical pathology is histopathology.

For some specimens, such as cardiac valves, a careful gross examination and description are infinitely superior to the examination of a random microscopic section. In many cases, an inadequate gross dissection and sampling will invalidate the microscopic interpretation.

Complicated specimens demand experience and knowledge in order to be dissected, described, and sampled adequately.

SURGICAL PATHOLOGY GROSS ROOM

The size and features of the surgical pathology gross room depend on the number of specimens, number of staff pathologists and residents, and type of institution. The gross room described in the following paragraphs is modeled after a large laboratory in an academic institution, but many of the requirements also apply to laboratories in small hospitals.

First of all, the room should be large enough to permit the simultaneous work of all the pathologists assigned to gross activities; it should be well illuminated and properly ventilated. We have been appalled at the number of pathology departments throughout the country that have woefully inadequate gross room facilities, some consisting merely of a table, a chair, a cutting board, a sink, and a shelf cornered between a cryostat and a secretarial desk.

Each dissection area should contain the following:

1. A cutting board placed inside a metal box designed in such a fashion that all the fluids will flow directly into the sink.
2. Shelves for specimen containers.
3. Ready access to a sink with hot and cold water
4. Ready access to formalin
5. Dictation equipment, preferably actuated by a pedal
6. Box of instruments, including heavy and small scissors, different sized smooth and toothed forceps, a malleable probe, a scalpel handle, disposable blades, a long knife, and pins for attaching specimens to a cork surface
7. Box with cassettes and labels

In addition, the gross room should contain the following central equipment:

1. A large formalin container—a very convenient arrangement consists of the suspension of a large container from the ceiling, with formalin pumped into it with a mechanical pump and the fixative delivered to the individual dissection areas by a tubing system ending in faucets.
2. Containers with other fixatives, with instructions on how to mix them at the time of use
3. Photographic facilities for black and white, color, and polaroid photographs and for photocopies
4. A self-contained X-ray unit (such as fixation)
5. Large refrigerator
6. Small refrigerator (e.g. for electron microscopy fixatives, photographic film)
7. Band saw—preferably one designed for use in butcher shops rather than those used by carpenters
8. Balances—one of large capacity for regular specimens and a delicate balance of small specimens, such as parathyroid glands.
9. Electrically driven, commercial meat cutter—results in excellent cross sections of solid specimens for demonstration and photographic purposes
10. Dissecting microscope
11. X-ray viewbox
12. Large sink for the dissection of large specimens (such as amputation)

13. Tissue procurement/tissue bank facilities—includes desk space, hood-enclosed cutting board, computer terminal, equipment and supplies for freezing specimens, freezer(s), and refrigerator.

FIXATION

Of the many fixatives that have been proposed, 10% buffered formalin remains the best compromise under most circumstances. It is inexpensive, the tissue can remain in it for prolonged periods without deterioration, the tissue can remain in it for prolonged periods without deterioration, as it is compatible with most special stains. "Pure" formalin is a concentrated (40%) solution of the gas formaldehyde in water. Thus a 10% formalin solution represents a 4% solution of the gas.

Zenker's is an excellent fixative, one of the best that has ever been devised for light microscopic work, but it is expensive, requires careful disposal of the mercury, and necessitates meticulous attention to fixation times and washing procedures to remove the precipitates of mercury.

Bouin's fixative has been especially recommended for testicular biopsies, but we have found that Zenker's fluid results in almost identical preparations.

Carnoy's fixative is a mixture that contains chloroform. Thus at the same time that it fixes the tissues, it dissolves most of the fat.

A fixative suitable for both light and electron microscopic examination ("universal fixative") is also available. It is made of mixture of 4% commercial paraformaldehyde and 1% glutaraldehyde in a neutral buffer. It is a convenient fixative to use, but it is less desirable than fixing the tissue immediately after it is excised in the corresponding fixatives for light and electron microscopy.

The volume of fixative should be at least ten times that of the tissue. The container should have an opening large enough so that the tissue can be removed easily after it has been hardened by the fixation. The fixative should surround the specimen on all slides. Large specimens that float on a fixative should be covered by a thick layer of gauze. In cases of large, flat, heavy specimens that rest on the bottom of the containers, the gauze should be placed between the container bottom and the specimen.

The fixation can be carried out at room temperature or, in the case of large specimens, at 4 °C (*see* the following discussion). Tissue should not be frozen once it has been placed in the fixative solution, for a peculiar ice crystal distortion will result. The freezing point of a 10% formalin solution is –3 °C.

GENERAL PRINCIPLES OF GROSS EXAMINATION

Proper identification and orientation of the specimen are always important and may be imperative for the adequate pathologic evaluation of a case. An unlabeled specimen should never be processed; if the biopsy is received in the laboratory without identification, the physician who performed the procedure or, in his absence, one of the assistants should be called to identify and label the specimen. A properly completed surgical pathology requisition form containing the patient's identification, age, and sex; essential clinical data; operation; surgical findings; and tissue submitted should accompany every specimen.

If there are difficulties with orientation of the specimen, the surgeon should be contacted and cooperation requested in identifying the position, anatomic landmarks, surgical margins, and any other structure of significance.

Surgeons should be instructed to submit to the pathology laboratory all the material that they have removed, not selected portions from it. The specimen, especially, if small, should be handled on a clean cutting board, using spotless, clean instruments. The problem of contamination of a specimen with a fragment from another (the "floater" or "cutting board metastasis") is one of the major catastrophes that can occur in the pathology laboratory because it can lead to irreparable mistakes.

The first step is a general inspection of the specimen, with identification of all of its normal and abnormal components. He should place the specimen on the cutting board in an anatomic position and record at this point the following information: (1) type of specimen, (2) structures included, (3) dimensions, (4) weight, (5) shape, and (6) color. This is also the time to identify the surgical margins in order to preserve them in subsequent steps and eventually study them microscopically. The pathologist should keep in mind that in many surgical excisions, the surgeon already knows the microscopic diagnosis of the lesion, and he is now interested in other information, such as extent of the lesion, invasion of neighboring structures, presence of tumor at the surgical margins, vascular invasion, and lymph node metastases. If a surgical margin is located, the accumulation of these data requires careful and sometimes tedious, but always rewarding, work.

Before the dissection of the specimen is begun, the advisability of taking gross photographs of the external surface should be considered. While this is a good practice for documentation purposes.

Three situations may arise during dissection of a surgical specimen:

1. It may be necessary to separate each of its main components in the fresh state, such as in a radical neck dissection.

2. It may be necessary to remove only some components (such as the regional lymph nodes) and leave the rest of the specimen as a single piece.

3. It may be better to fix the entire specimen as a block. This can be achieved in several ways, depending on the size, shape, and presence or absence of a cavity in the specimen. Small specimens without particularly thick areas are simply placed in a fixative at room temperature. Larger specimens that cannot be satisfactorily injected (such as a radical resection of a soft tissue tumor or a nephrectomy specimen) are better fixed overnight in a refrigerator at 4 °C to slow the autolytic process. Hollow specimens are either opened fresh or else fixed simultaneously from the outside and the inside. The latter is achieved either by injecting the cavity with formalin by syringe or catheter or by packing the cavity with gauze or cotton impregnated with formalin. Cystic lesions (such as ovarian cystadenomas) can be injected with formalin after the original fluid has been removed. Multilocular cysts require individual injection of the larger cavities, combined with fixation of the specimen block at 4 °C.

As a general rule, when a specimen is sliced, and assuming that several of the slices show similar features, it is advisable to leave one of the best slices intact for possible photography, gross demonstration, or display as a museum specimen. Under no circumstances should any portion of a specimen be discarded before the case is signed out. Actually, it is advisable to save the wet tissue for a minimum of 2 or 3 months.

SPECIMEN THERAPY

Documentation of the gross features of a surgical specimen is best achieved by taking one or several gross photographs of the lesion, in the form of either color transparencies or black-and-white prints. Methods for recording photographically gross specimens consist in taking black-and-white or color prints with analog or digital cameras. These images can also be stored electronically.

1. A common mistake is to take a photograph of the external surface of the intact tumor (which is often meaningless, other than providing some information on overall size and configuration) but forgetting to take a photograph of the cut surface, which is usually much more informative.

2. Some consideration should be given to what is the best view of the lesion before the picture is taken. If a specimen is cut in two, it is better to photograph one half rather than both halves of a partially cut specimen.

3. Preparation and trimming of the specimen are important. This includes removing fat and other unnecessary tissue around the lesion, opening ducts and vessels, and trimming fat around the latter structures.

4. The background should be spotlessly clean, be kept to a minimum, have no texture, and be illuminated. For color photographs, a gray-toned neutral-intensity color is preferable (we use a light blue). The use of drapes, sponges, and gauzes is to be discouraged.

5. Rulers should be used only when reference to size is important. They should be as unobstrusive as possible, always in the metric systems, without advertisements or other distractions, clean, clearly legible, and placed in such a way as to allow a quick determination of the measurements of the lesion. They should be of adequate size and be kept in focus by raising or lowering them according to the height of the specimen.

6. Knife marks in the cut surface should be avoided by using sharp instruments and by cutting the specimens with a continuous, slow motion of the hand.

7. The specimen should be properly oriented, centered, and framed. A common mistake is to use only half or less of the field of a photograph. An increase in magnification improves the resolution of detail in the specimen without the loss of any important information.

8. Whenever possible, normal structures should be included in the photograph to serve as a frame of reference for the lesion.

9. Objects such as hands, forceps, probes, scissors, and paper clips are distracting and should generally be avoided.

10. Specimen identification by the use of labels on top of the lesion is distracting. It is better to write the pathology number on the frame than to include it in the projected photograph.

11. Reflective glare (specular reflections) should be avoided by properly placing the illumination system, by turning off the room lights, by blotting the cut section of the specimen with a guaze, and if necessary, by using diffusion screens.

12. The proper exposure can be determined with a light meter by trial and error. It is always advisable to take several photographs of a lesion, using slightly different exposures.

13. For specimens of substantial height, the lens aperture should be as small as possible (f-stop of 16 or greater) to increase the depth of field.

14. Heightened image clarity and contrast can be obtained by the use of ultraviolet illumination.

SPECIMEN RADIOGRAPHY

Radiographic examination of surgical specimens sometimes provides important information. Specimens particularly suitable for this type of examination include bone lesions, calcified soft tissue masses, breast biopsies and excisions (especially if they had been studied by mammography), cardiac valves, and lymph nodes groups in which a lymphangiogram had been taken. Areas of calcification (particularly important in breast biopsies) can be detected even in the paraffin blocks if the cassettes are made of plastic or some other radiolucent material. Radiopaque foreign bodies (such as metal clips) can be spotted easily.

SAMPLING FOR HISTOLOGIC EXAMINATION

Tissues submitted for histology must not be more than 3 mm thick and not larger than the dimensions of the cassette used; otherwise they will not be adequately infiltrated by paraffin. Adipose tissue must be cut even thinner. Overfilling of the cassette should be avoided, or the tissue will not be infiltrated. Suture material, metal clips, and other foreign bodies should be removed from the tissues before putting them in cassettes, or the microtone knives will be damaged. If the fragments are very small, it is advisable to stain them with hematoxylin and mercurochrome before putting them in the cassette to facilitate their identification by the histotechnologist.

Most specimens from solid tissues are cut in the form of pieces measuring 10 to 15 mm on the sides and 2 to 3 mm in thickness; the histotechnologist will orient them in a flat position in the paraffin block. If one side shows a given feature better than the opposite side, the pathologist can indicate this with India ink on the side opposite the one to be cut. The pathologist can help the histotechnologist by showing him the specimen before putting it in the cassette, by embedding it in paraffin himself, or by surrounding it with a material that will keep it in the desired position during the processing steps. We use for this purpose a solution of 3% agar in distilled water, kept in a viscous fluid state at 60°C. The specimen is kept on edge with small forceps on top of a glass slide while 1 or 2 drops of the agar solution are applied to it. Once this solidifies (it should take less than a minute), it is detached from the slide with a sharp blade and transferred to the cassette. Further description of this technique is given in Appendix H.

To ensure adequate sampling, multiple microscopic sections ("various levels" or VL) should be requested for some specimens at the time that the gross description is dictated. This includes biopsies from the respiratory tract, gastrointestinal tract, bladder, lymph nodes, and bone marrow; all needle and punch biopsies; and in general, all specimens measuring 3 mm or less.

GUIDELINES FOR HANDLING THE MOST COMMON AND IMPORTANT SURGICAL SPECIMENS

In order to achieve a certain consistency in the way the specimens are handled in the gross room, it is important for a manual of procedures to be available to the person performing the gross examination to assist him in dissecting the specimen, describing it, taking the appropriate sections for microscopic examination, and performing whatever other additional tasks may be required depending on the nature of the case.

3

Special Techniques in Surgical Pathology

The mainstay of surgical pathology is (and is likely to remain for a long time) the examination of the specimens following fixation in formalin, processing in graded alcohols and xylene or other solvents, embedding in paraffin, cutting of sections with a microtome, and staining with hematoxylin–eosin (H&E).

In the H&E technique, hematoxylin staining of nuclei is followed by counterstaining of cytoplasms and various extracellular materials by eosin. Hematoxylin is extracted from the bark of a tropical wood, *Haematoxylum campechianum* ('Bloody red bark tree' from Campeche, Mexico). In order to function as a nuclear stain, it needs to be oxidized ('ripened') to the purple dye hematein and provided with a net positive charge by combining it ('chelating') with a metallic salt ('mordant'). Eosin is an anionic xanthene dye that combines electrostatically with various cytoplasmic components and with tissue such as collagen or muscle, the latter in an amphoteric manner.

This technique has proved one of the most durables in medicine and has remained essentially unchanged—except for automation and time compression of some of the steps—for over half a century. This may be due in part to a certain resistance to change that has been attributed to the practitioners of pathology.

Considerable Advantages

It is relatively quick, inexpensive, suitable for most situations, and comparatively easy to master. Most important, it allows an accurate microscopic diagnosis of the large majority of specimens sent to the laboratory.

The special techniques that have been found most helpful in diagnostic pathology over the years are discussed in this chapter.

Special Stains

Of the hundreds of 'special' stains listed in the classic texts dealing with histologic techniques, the surgical pathologist will find a relatively small minority to be of real diagnostic utility at present. This is especially true since the advent of immunohistochemistry, which has rendered many of them obsolete.

Those most commonly used at present are the following:

Periodic acid–Schiff (PAS) stain. Substances containing vicinal glycol groups or their amino or alkylamino derivatives are oxidized by periodic acid to form dialdehydes, which combine with the Schiff reagent to form an insoluble magenta compound. This stain therefore demonstrates glycogen (in a specific fashion, when used with a diastase-digested control) and neutral mucosubstances, outlines basement membranes, and makes evident most types of fungi and parasites. As a trivia, one might add that it is also useful for the demonstration of the intra-cytoplasmic crystals in alveolar soft part sarcoma.

Stains for Microorganisms

These include techniques for gram-positive and gram-negative bacteria, acid-fast mycobacteria, fungi, and parasites. The gram stain allows the separation of bacteria into those that retain the crystal violet–iodine complex (gram positive) and those that are decolorized by alcohol or acetone treatment and counterstained by either safranin or fuchsin. Acid fastness depends on the high lipid content (mycolic acids and long-chain fatty acids) in the cell walls of mycobacteria, which confer to the cell the ability to complex basic dyes (such as carbolfuchsin) and to retain them following strong decoloration with acid–alcohol. The techniques in this group most used are Brown and Brenn (B&B; as a modification of the gram stain), Ziehl–Neelsen (for acid-fast organisms), Grocott hexamine–silver (for fungi and Pneumocystis), PAS (for fungi, amoebae, and Trichomonas), and Dieterle or one of its modifications (for Helicobacter, Legionella, and the organisms of syphilis and Lyme disease).

Argentaffin and Argyrophilic Stains

The argentaffin reaction depends on the presence in the tissue of a substance, often of the phenolic group (such as catecholamines or indolamines), that reduces silver (and other metallic) salts; we generally use the Fontana–Masson technique in paraffin-embedded material. In the argyrophilic reaction, an extraneous reducing agent such as hydroquinone or formalin is added; we generally employ the unmodified Grimelius technique and prefer to use it in Bouin fixed material whenever available. Others have found the Churukian-Schenk's modification to give better results.

Silver Stains

They are mainly used for the identification of neuroendocrine cells and their tumors, but also for the demonstration of reticulin fibers, melanin, and calcium.

Amyloid Stains

The mysteriously named Congo red followed by examination with both standard and polarized light (the notorious apple green birefringence) is regarded as the most reliable and practical technique to detect amyloid. It should be realized, however, that the stain does not have chemical specificity, being dependent upon an arrangement of the molecule in an antiparallel beta-pleated sheet. It should also be noted that nonamyloid-related green birefringence can occur as a result of excess dye retained in the tissue and to other technical factors.

Reticulin Stains

Reticulin stains demonstrate both 'reticular fibers' and basement membrane material. Reticular fibers consist of very thin fibers of mainly type III collagen, which are widespread in connective tissue throughout the body. Basement membranes are largely composed of type IV collagen and laminin. In both instances it appears that the adsorption of silver stains and their PAS positivity are due to a coating of bound proteoglycans. Reticular fibers and reticulin stains should not be equated to reticulum cells, a common misconception. The latter term refers to cells (generally of the accessory immune system, also called dendritic cells) in which the 'reticulum' or network is formed not by extracellular material but by thin, complex cytoplasmic prolongations.

Traditionally, the main applications of silver-based reticulin stains (such as Gomori, Wilder, and Gordon and Sweet) in tumor pathology have been in distinguishing: (1) epithelial from nonepithelial neoplasms; (2) various mesenchymal neoplasms from each other; and (3) *in situ* from invasive carcinoma. In general, foci of carcinoma have reticulin around the tumor nests but not between the individual cells, whereas in most sarcomas and large cell lymphomas the silver-positive material separates single cells. The striking contrast between the two patterns can be readily appreciated by comparing the epithelial and mesenchymal components of a synovial sarcoma. In tumors of endothelial cells, the reticulin that identifies the vessel wall (rather than the one which coats the individual tumor cells) is seen on the outside of the neoplastic population, whereas the reverse is true in tumors of pericytes or vascular smooth muscle cells. In typical cases of leiomyosarcoma the reticulin wraps individual cells completely, whereas in typical cases of malignant peripheral nerve sheath tumor it runs in parallel to the spindle tumor cells without surrounding them at the poles. Reticulin stains have also been used to distinguish ovarian granulosa cell tumors (in which the fibers are scanty and surrounding groups of cells) from fibrothecomas (in which they surround individual tumor cells). Unfortunately, these patterns are well in evidence only in classic cases of these respective entities, i.e. those which are already easily diagnosable with H&E techniques. In the controversial cases, reticulin stains are likely to provide results that are far from conclusive, to the point that we have found them of very limited utility.

Trichrome Stains

In the trichrome methods, such as those devised by Masson, van Gieson, and Mallory, phosphotungstic or phosphomolybdic acid is used in combination with several anionic dyes. The main value of this group of stains is in the evaluation of the type and amount of extracellular material. The three tissue structures demonstrated by the three component dyes are nuclei, cytoplasm, and extracellular collagen, respectively. It is not generally realized that the only component of all trichrome stains having some degree of specificity is that provided by the phosphotungstic or phosphomolybdic acid, which stains the collagen fibers; everything else is background staining, no better from the point of view of specificity than what is obtained with H&E.

Phosphotungstic Acid–Hematoxylin (PTAH) Stain

This particular variant of trichrome stain has been traditionally used for the demonstration of intracytoplasmic filaments, such as those present in muscle and glial cells.

Stains for Hemosiderin (Perls), Melanin (Fontana–Masson), and Calcium (von Kossa)

In the Perls technique for hemosiderin, hydrochloric acid splits off the protein bound to the iron, allowing the potassium ferrocyanide to combine specifically with the ferric iron to form ferric ferrocyanide (Prussian blue). In the Fontana–Masson method for melanin, an ammoniacal silver solution is used without a reducing bath. Only substances capable of reducing directly silver salts (i.e. argentaffin) such as melanin are demonstrated. In the von Kossa method for calcium, silver is substituted for calcium in calcium salts; this silver salt is then reduced to black metallic silver by the use of light or a photographic developer.

Stains for Neutral Lipids

Most of these stains are based on the principle that the colored compounds used are more soluble in the tissue lipids than in their own solvent. Actually, these compounds do not qualify as dyes in the conventional sense, in that they contain no auxochromic groups but are chromogens. Oil red O is the one most commonly employed. A limitation of fat stains is the fact that they cannot be performed in paraffin-embedded material because of the fat solubilizing properties of xylene and other clearing materials used for processing. In tumor pathology, the utility of fat stains is minimal and largely limited to the inconsequential distinction between fibroma and thecoma in the ovary, support for the diagnosis of renal cell carcinoma and sebaceous gland tumors of skin, and identification of lipid-rich carcinoma in various organs. Despite ingrained notions to the contrary, fat stains are of little if any use for the diagnosis of liposarcoma; some liposarcomas contain a little or no stainable fat, whereas several types of nonadipose tissue neoplasms can contain considerable amounts.

Mucin Stains

Mucin is the traditional term used for a large group of macro-molecules containing an acidic group, which is divided into two major categories: The epithelial O-glycoproteins (membrane-bound or secreted) composed of a protein core and a sialic acid-containing carbohydrate moiety (whether sulfated or not) and the stromal glycosaminoglycans, which contain hyaluronic acid and which also can be sulfated. Historically, the term 'mucin' has been used for the former category, whereas the latter substance has been usually referred to as 'myxoid' (hence the term pseudomyxoma for a lesion that may appear myxoid, i.e. stromal, but is really epithelial, i.e. mucinous). The combination of Alcian blue and PAS is probably the best 'pan-mucin' stain, since it demonstrates mucosubstances of neutral, slightly acidic, and highly acidic types. Enzymatic pretreatment will show whether the acidic groups are made of sialic acid (digestible with sialidase), hyaluronic acid (digestible with hyaluronidase), or sulfated groups (digestible with neither). Several stains are available for the specific demonstration of highly acidic mucins. These include Alcian blue performed at pH 1.0, colloidal iron, high iron-diamine, and the classic Mayer mucicarmine. The abnormalities in mucin secretion sometimes present in carcinomas (usually because of incomplete carbohydrate synthesis) can be surmised from the mucin stains but require more sophisticated techniques for their specific identification. Mucin stains are also used to classify gastric incomplete metaplasia into subtypes (sialomucin- and sulfomucin-containing) having supposedly different malignant potentials. It should be noted that all of the mucin stains mentioned above demonstrate the carbohydrate component of these glycoproteins. Lately, immunohistochemical identification of the protein core of the same molecules (MUC) is providing a different type of separation of these molecules, which may be of greater diagnostic significance.

Giemsa Stain

The most spectacular results with Giemsa and other Romanovsky-type stains are obtained with alcohol-fixed smears. However, reasonably good preparations can also be achieved in paraffin-embedded material, provided one is very scrupulous with the technique and fastidious with the source of the reagents. The technique is most useful for the demonstration of various hematolymphoid elements (including mast cells) and microorganisms.

Elastic Fibers

Weigert-type techniques are reasonably specific for elastin and are regarded by many as the method of choice for the demonstration of these extracellular fibers. However, the Verhoeff–van Gieson (VVG) stain is more popular because it is quick and outlines the elastic fibers with a strong black color. Both techniques are usually set against the esthetically pleasant trichrome background provided by the van Gieson stain.

Myelin Stains

Luxol fast blue is the nonimmunohistochemical method of choice for the demonstration of myelin. It is based on the strong affinity of the copper phthalocyanine dye for the phospholipids and choline bases of myelin.

Formaldehyde-induced Fluorescence

This is a very special type of technique, remarkably sensitive for the demonstration of catecholamines and indolamines but requiring rather costly and cumbersome equipment as originally described. A modified version as applied to touch preparations has made it more accessible to the practicing pathologist, but it is rarely used at the present time. It is based on the principle that biogenic amines subjected to formaldehyde vapors produced by heating the polymer paraformaldehyde form highly fluorescent derivatives

Enzyme Histochemistry

After a period of enthusiasm in the 1950s and 1960s for the use of enzyme histochemical techniques in pathology they fell in general disuse as far as diagnostic applications were concerned. This was due to the complexity of the techniques, the need for fresh material, and the relative nonspecificity of most of the reactions. In the present time, the enzyme histochemical methods most commonly used for diagnostic purposes are those for skeletal muscle-related enzymes (for the study of myopathies), acetylcholinesterase (for the diagnosis of Hirschsprung disease), and chloroacetate esterase (for the identification of cells of the myeloid series and mast cells). The latter, known as Leder's technique, benefits from the fact that chloroacetate esterase is one of the few enzymes that resists the effects of formalin fixation and paraffin embedding. Another enzyme that can be demonstrated following routine procedures is acid phosphatase.

A plastic embedding technique following paraformaldehyde fixation has been described that combines preservation of various enzymes with excellent morphologic detail. Another enzyme histochemical technique with diagnostic connotations is the DOPA reaction for cells of the melanocytic series. It depends on the presence of the enzyme tyrosinase and requires the use of fresh tissue. A modified version of the technique allows the demonstration of the precipitation product in paraffin-embedded material.

Tissue Culture

The pioneer work of Margaret Murray, Arthur Purdy Stout, and Luciano Ozzello at Columbia-Presbyterian Hospital in New York City showed that some histogenetic clues could be obtained from the examination of primary cultures of human tumors such as thymoma, synovial sarcoma, rhabdomyosarcoma, and hemangiopericytoma. The concepts of the existence of fibrous mesothelioma and fibrous histiocytoma were to a large extent based on tissue culture observations by these investigators.

The rationale for the diagnostic application of tissue culture in human tumors is based on the observation that tumor cells can express features of differentiation *in vitro* that are not exhibited or not appreciable *in vivo*.

It should be apparent that cells grown in culture can be studied with any of the modern tools such as immunohistochemistry, electron microscopy, ultrastructural immunohistochemistry, cytogenetics, and molecular biologic techniques.

Quantitative Methods (histometry)

Objective measurement of microscopic features has been advocated for decades as a method to make more reproducible and 'scientific' the practice of histopathology, but it is only relatively recently that technical advances in computing technology have rendered this procedure suitable for diagnostic and prognostic determinations in surgical pathology. Traditionally the measurements have been made from photographs, from projected images, or by the use of eyepiece graticules. Currently, semiautomatic or fully automated image analyzers are employed.

At present, the method is also applied with increasing frequency to various aspects of tumor pathology, such as determination of DNA ploidy (in Feulgen-stained preparations): Proliferative index (after staining of the sections with MIB-1 (Ki-67) or analogous markers), nuclear grading, dysplasia grading, hormone receptor status, and HER2/neu status. In the case of DNA ploidy and proliferative index evaluations, image analysis has been proved to be as accurate as flow cytometry, and clearly superior to it in some specific situations, such as when the amount of tissue is scanty or when the ratio of tumor to non-neoplastic elements is low.

Electron Microscopy

The main applications of electron microscopy to diagnostic pathology are in the fields of renal and tumor pathology. In tumor pathology, ultrastructural examinations have proved very useful in determining the histogenesis (or differentiation) of various tumors but, unfortunately, have not shown consistent differences between reactive conditions, benign tumors, and malignant tumors of the same cell type.

The best chance for electron microscopy to be of utility is when the pathologist has already formulated a definite differential diagnosis between two or three entities at the light microscopic level and examines the tissue ultrastructurally searching specifically for the markers to be expected in each of those entities.

The limitations of electron microscopy can be summarized as follows:

1. Sampling, wherein only a small proportion of the neoplasm can be studied.
2. Paucity of truly specific ultrastructural features, since the number of organelles or other structures that are exclusive of a cell or tissue type is very small.
3. Possible misinterpretation of entrapped non-neoplastic elements as belonging to the tumor. Admittedly, this possibility exists with any technique, but it is particularly noticeable with electron microscopy because of the difficulties in evaluating spatial relationships in a small tissue sample.

Immunohistochemistry

Briefly stated, immunohistochemistry is the application of immunologic principles and techniques to demonstrate molecules in cells and tissues. The original method, brilliantly conceived by Coons, consisted of labeling with a fluorescent probe an antibody raised in rabbits and searching for it (and therefore for the antigen against which the antibody was directed) in tissue sections examined under a fluorescent microscope following incubation. The technical improvements that supervened in subsequent years have been responsible for these methods becoming a staple of the histopathology laboratory.

Many immunohistochemical detection techniques are available, the ones most commonly used at present being the polymer-based method and the biotin–avidin immunoenzymatic technique. In the latter procedure, the high affinity of avidin for biotin is used to couple the peroxidase label to the primary antibody.

Various methods for increasing the sensitivity of the procedure have been devised. Their aim is to expose antigenic sites (epitopes) that may otherwise be unexposed ('masked'), hence their generic designation as 'antigen-unmasking' or 'antigen-retrieving' techniques. They include digestion with a variety of proteolytic enzymes, and treatment with wet heat obtained with a microwave oven, water bath, pressure cooker.

There is probably no other method that has so revolutionized the field during the past 50 years as the immunohistochemical technique. The advantages are obvious: Remarkable sensitivity and specificity, applicability to routinely processed material (even if stored for long periods), and feasibility of an accurate correlation with the traditional morphologic parameters. It is compatible with most of the fixatives currently in use and is feasible even in decalcified material or in previously stained microscopic sections. It is sometimes positive even in totally necrotic material. It can also be adapted to cytologic preparations and to electron microscopy.

A quick labeling method (<7 min) has been devised for its possible use in intraoperative consultation, such as evaluation of sentinel lymph nodes. A variety of instruments for the automation of immunohistology have become standard in pathology laboratories.

False-negative results in immunohistochemistry can occur when:

1. An antibody is inappropriate, denatured, or used at the wrong concentration.

2. There is loss of antigen through autolysis and/or diffusion. This factor plays a much larger role with some antigens (such as factor VIII-related antigen) than with others (such as actin). It should be remembered that antigens can continue to leak out after fixation; therefore, it is always preferable to perform the stains using the original paraffin block rather than tissue left in formalin for long periods.

3. Presence of antigen is at a density below the level of detection with the reagents and techniques used, because of either minimal production or excessive release.

Because of the existence of all these factors, an apparently negative immunohistochemical result should not be used to rule out a diagnosis even in the presence of a positive built-in control, especially if such a diagnosis is strongly suggested by the clinical and morphologic features.

False positive results, which are even more dangerous, can result from a variety of causes:

1. Cross-reactivity of the antibody with antigens different from the one being sought.

2. Nonspecific binding of the antibody to the tissue.

3. Presence of endogenous peroxidase in—or avidity for the avidin–biotin complex by—some cellular elements (depending on the immunohistochemical detection system being used).

4. Entrapment of normal tissues by the tumor cells. This problem, which also exists in H&E-stained sections, is amplified through the great sensitivity of the technique.

5. Release of proteins from the cytoplasm of normal cells invaded by the tumor, with subsequent permeation of the interstitium and nonspecific absorption (and possibly phagocytosis) by the tumor cells. Perhaps in some cases this phenomenon—which is the most treacherous of them all—represents an artifact developed after the removal of the tissue, but in most instances it is probably occurring already *in vivo*.

Flow Cytometry

The technique of flow cytometry consists of the measurement of various parameters while a suspension of cells flows through a beam of light past stationary detectors. The instrument focuses hydrodynamically a cell suspension in a sample chamber and passes single cells through a light source, usually a laser. The light scattered at various angles by the cells is registered by detectors and converted to electronic signals, which are then digitized, stored, and analyzed by the computer to produce a histogram. This technique allows the analysis of 5000–10000 cells per second. Cellular features that can be evaluated with flow cytometry include cell size, cytoplasmic granularity, cell viability, cell cycle time (S-phase fraction), DNA content (DNA ploidy), surface marker phenotype, and enzyme content. Technical advances now allow for several parameters to be evaluated simultaneously.

Other Methods for Analysis of Cell Proliferation

In addition to flow cytometry (S-phase fraction), several other methods are available for the evaluation of the degree of cellular proliferation in tumor tissue.

The older and still widely used method is mitotic count in routinely processed sections, the standard figure employed being the number of mitoses in a certain number (usually 10–50) of consecutive 'high-power' fields (usually defined as the combination of 10× eyepiece and 40× objective). The method has found its most useful application in the evaluation of mesenchymal neoplasms (particularly uterine smooth muscle tumors), breast carcinoma, neuroblastoma, and GIST, either by itself or as a key component of the grading system. Despite its apparent objectivity, it is subject to considerable variations depending on the thickness of the section, fields chosen, type of microscope used, delay in fixation time, and observer's variability in the identification of mitotic figures.

In our opinion, an even greater drawback of this technique as currently used is the blatantly inaccurate and archaic nature of the denominator used (i.e. a microscopic 'field'). A considerably more accurate and rational way of making this determination would be by expressing the number of mitotic figures as a function of the percentage of tumor cells, irrespective of the number of non-neoplastic cells and intercellular material present, as investigators counting nuclei labeled with thymidine have always done.

Another time-honored method for evaluating cell proliferation consists in counting nuclei in S-phase (DNA synthesis) following *in vitro* thymidine labeling, paraffin embedding, and auto-radiography. The standard determination of the thymidine labeling index (TLI) is done by counting 2000 tumor nuclei.

Microspectrophotometric analysis is performed by staining tissue sections obtained from paraffin-embedded material with the Feulgen reaction (which is specific for DNA) and determining the DNA content (expressed in arbitrary units) in a micro-spectrophotometer using a single wavelength of 560 μm. This tedious technique has been largely replaced by flow cytometry, but it is still being used by some authors.

Cell proliferation can also be investigated with immuno-histochemical techniques by staining for nuclear antigens related to cell growth and division, and searching for them visually under the microscope or with the help of an image analyser.

Ki-S1 is another proliferation marker that is detectable after formalin fixation and paraffin embedding, and which has been found to be identical with topoisomerase IIa. It functions as a cofactor for polymerase delta during the DNA synthesis phase of the cell cycle.

Nucleolar organizer region (NOR) evaluation is another indicator of cell proliferation, although of a very different kind. First described as weakly staining chromatinic regions around which nucleoli reorganize during telophase, NORs are now known to contain ribosomal genes (as shown by *in situ* hybridization) and a number of acidic proteins that have a high affinity for silver (AgNOR proteins). The latter feature has been effectively used for the rapid identification of NORs in light microscopic sections using a simple one-step silver technique. NORs appear as black dots of metallic silver, about 0.5–1 μm in diameter, localized within secondary constrictions of metaphase chromosomes or within nuclei.

Cytogenetics

Karyotypic analysis of human tumors, considered in the past a relatively unrewarding exercise because of the seemingly random and secondary nature of the alterations, has proved to be a powerful tool for the study of tumors, both in terms of contributing to the definition of the various entities and in providing clues to the molecular mechanisms involved in their pathogenesis.

The detection of nonrandom or specific chromosome abnor-malities—such as deletions, amplifications, inversions, and translocations—has been particularly successful in the fields of leukemias and lymphomas, germ cell tumors, pediatric tumors, and mesenchymal neoplasms but less so in carcinomas. These are further discussed in the respective chapters.

Because of the labor-intensive, time-consuming nature of this analysis and the requirement for fresh tissues, new techniques have been sought for detecting numerical and structural chromosomal abnormalities in a faster and more efficient fashion. One such technique, interphase cytogenetics, is discussed in a subsequent section. Another method is comparative genomic hybridization (CGH). In this procedure, chromosomes are competitively hybridized with two differentially labeled genomic DNAs (one from the test case and the other from a reference case). These, when examined with fluorescence microscopy, show the chromosomal locations of copy number changes in DNA sequences between the two complements (i.e. between tumor and normal DNA). CGH can be applied to fresh-frozen specimens, cell lines, and also DNA extracted from formalin-fixed, paraffin-embedded material. It should be noted that CGH can only detect gain or loss of chromosomes and chromosome segments, but not balanced chromosomal translocations. An ingenious technique has been developed to correlate the microscopic phenotype of solid tumors with their genotype by using universal DNA amplification, CGH, and interphase cytogenetics in formalin-fixed, paraffin-embedded material.

Molecular Pathology

The revolutionary advances made in molecular biology are having a major impact on the practice of surgical pathology. Indeed, they have the potential to change the practice in a way that no other techniques ever had before. Advances are occurring at such a rate that it has become very difficult to capture them in a book format, even if highly specialized. Therefore, only a general and, I am afraid, superficial overview of the field will be given, interspersed with some personal reflections.

A gene is a segment of DNA containing the codes for the amino acid sequence of a polypeptide and the regulatory sequences that control its expression. The coding DNA sequences (exons) of a gene are often interrupted by noncoding sequences (introns). After translation into messenger RNA, the noncoding nucleotides are removed during RNA splicing. Gene expression is regulated by many factors, such as the gene promoter, transcription factors and DNA methylation. In addition, microRNA, a newly recognized class of small RNA (usually 21–26 nucleotides long) inactivates specific messenger RNAs in a sequence-specific manner.

Filter Hybridization

In this form of nucleic acid hybridization, target DNA is extracted from tissues and immobilized on filters made of nitrocellulose or nylon. This can be done directly as 'dot blots' or after the performance of restriction enzyme digestion, size fractionation by gel electrophoresis, and subsequent transfer into the filter (Southern blot, named after its inventor, EM Southern). This is followed by hybridizing the bound nucleic acid to a labeled probe, masking, and detecting the bound probe. Dot blot hybridization is used when size fractionation of nucleic acid is not required, such as detection of DNA of specific microorganisms. Procedures analogous to Southern blotting but involving size fractionation of RNA or protein are known as Northern and Western blotting, respectively (a pun on Southern's last name). Filter hybridization is best done using fresh tissue. Attempts have been made to develop a fixative suitable for routine work and also capable of preserving as much as possible the integrity of the nucleic acids.

The filter hybridization method is ideally suited for the identification and analysis of the following genomic alterations: (1) gene rearrangements; (2) gene amplifications; (3) gene deletions; and (4) point mutations. It is a powerful technique, but it suffers from a number of technical disadvantages, such as slow turn around time, the need for radioactive compounds (although nonisotopic detection methods are also available), and the susceptibility of the method to various artifacts. Therefore, alternative techniques have been developed, including those discussed in the following sections.

In situ Hybridization

In situ hybridization (ISH) consists of the detection of specific DNA or RNA sequences in tissue sections or cell preparations using a labeled complementary nucleic acid sequence or probe. Under the appropriate conditions, this probe will hybridize (through the establishment of hydrogen bonds) to the target DNA or RNA and be visualized by either radioactive (^{32}P, ^{125}I, ^{35}S, ^{3}H), nonradioactive (peroxidase, biotin, digoxigenin) or fluorochrome labels incorporated into the probe. The last type is commonly known as fluorescent in situ hybridization (FISH). Both the target and probe nucleic acid need to be single stranded for the hybridization to take place. The main probes currently in use for ISH are cloned RNA and DNA probes and synthetic oligonucleotide probes.

ISH has mainly been used for the detection of viral infections (such as HPV, EBV, and HIV), taking advantage of the ability of the technique to identify directly the viral genome within the infected cell. An advantage this offers over immunohistochemistry is that it can detect not only productive but also latent infections, as well as segregate the various virus subtypes, as in HPV. Also, in the area of infectious diseases, it has been found useful for the distinction among Aspergillus and other fungal species in tissue sections.

ISH has also been used to detect gene expression by neoplasms. One such use is the detection of messenger RNA for various peptide hormones, immunoglobulin light chains, and albumin. In many such cases, the technique proves successful when the immunohistochemical detection of the corresponding protein yields uninterpretable results. This is explained by the fact that diffusion of the proteins into the cells from the interstitial body fluids can render interpretation of immunohistochemical staining difficult if not impossible. On the other hand, positive staining for messenger RNA by ISH definitively indicates synthesis and the presence of the corresponding protein in the cells.

Increasingly, ISH is used for demonstration of various genetic alterations in tumors to aid in diagnosis and prognostication by the interphase cytogenetics concept.

ISH can be performed in conjunction with immunohisto-chemistry, combined with PCR (*in situ* PCR), or carried out at the electron microscopic level by the use of colloidal gold.

Interphase Cytogenetics

Interphase cytogenetics refers to the analysis of chromosomes in nondividing cells. As such, it is to be contrasted with the conventional chromosomal analysis performed in metaphase spreads. The latter depends on the presence of a suitable number of dividing cells in the sample, in order to allow the chromosomes to be counted and analyzed after the mitoses have been arrested in metaphase. This method, although proved highly successful under the right circumstances, has many important limitations. The specimen must be fresh, establishment of *in vitro* culture may be necessary, the dividing cell population may not be representative of the original sample, and the chromosomes may be of poor quality.

Interphase cytogenetics, which is notably free of these shortcomings, has become one of the most rapidly growing fields following the development of extremely sensitive detection methods and an ever-growing number of chromosome-specific DNA probes. FISH has proved particularly powerful because of its great sensitivity and rapidity, but fluorescence microscopy set-up is required and correlation with morphology is less than ideal. Chromogenic ISH (CISH) and silver ISH (SISH) are alternative methods whereby application of labeled probes followed by detection techniques results in color products visible under the light microscope, and thus permits better correlation of positive signals with morphology.

4

Maxilla and Mandible

In most respects, the microscopic features of the maxilla and mandible differ in no significant way from those of any other bones. Their peculiarity is derived from their close proximity to the mucosal surface of the oral cavity and the fact that they enclose the odontogenic apparatus, a highly specialized structure that gives rise to a large variety of malformative, inflammatory, and neoplastic conditions.

The odontogenic compartment is unique in the sense that it contains primitive embryonic structures from early fetal development to about 25 years of age. They have a combined ectodermal and mesodermal derivation; the mesodermal component has the added peculiarity that it originates from the neural crest (the so-called ectomesenchyme). The odontogenic development as seen in a tooth germ is a striking example of reciprocal inductive phenomena between two different types of tissue. The first is composed of an invagination of the ectodermally derived primitive oral cavity (dental lamina), which subsequently acquires a bell shape and develops along its inner (concave) aspects a layer of cuboidal to columnar cells, the ameloblasts, which are responsible for the secretion of enamel matrix. At this stage, it is also referred to as the enamel organ.

The second component, which is mesodermally derived and enclosed within the above described bell, is formed by the dental papilla, having initially the appearance of a loose stellate reticulum and later undergoing a maturation of its outer aspect that results in the emergence of odontoblasts. An increase in the cellularity of the dental papilla adjacent to the maturing ameloblastic (enamel-forming) epithelium leads to the formation of the dental sac or follicle, which is in turn responsible for the formation of a dense fibrous sheath enveloping the tooth known as periodontium. In addition, the inner cells of this sac become cementoblasts and deposit cement over the newly formed dentin, whereas the more peripheral cells of this structure are thought to become osteoblasts and to contribute to the production of alveolar bone.

The major extracellular components of the tooth are dentin, enamel, and cementum. Dentin is easily recognized because of its radially striated appearance caused by the presence of innumerable minute canals containing cytoplasmic processes from the odontoblasts. When these canals are absent, it may be difficult to distinguish between atypical poorly mineralized dentin (dentinoid) and osteoid. Enamel consists of thin rods or prisms that on cross section are separated by concentric lines. Cementum is very similar to bone in physicochemical characteristics and is indeed regarded as a special type of bundle bone. It may be cellular or acellular, and it is identified microscopically mainly because of its intense basophilia. When less than entirely typical, its distinction from conventional bone may become impossible. It must be recognized that cementum-like material may be encountered in parts of the skeletal system other than the maxilla or mandible, in which participation of odontogenic tissue would seem out of the question.

The presence of rounded, strongly basophilic cementicles within the periodontal ligament is a normal feature. It should not be misinterpreted as evidence of Paget disease, as it often is by the neophyte.

The dental pulp has a myxoid hypocellular appearance that is essentially identical to that of myxoma and that sometimes can be confused with it by the same neophyte. It differs from the latter grossly because of its most compact appearance and micro-scopically because a layer of odontoblasts may be recognizable at the periphery. Nests of odontogenic epithelium are normally found in the jaw and have the potential to develop into cysts or tumors. Those nests located in the alveolar mucosa and resulting from the breakup of the dental lamina are referred to as rests of Serres, whereas those embedded within the periodontium are known as rests of Malassez. Another source of cysts in this region is related to the breakdown of ectodermal lining cells during the union or fusion of the various embryonic processes of the region, through the formation of entrapped epithelium-lined nests.

The surgical pathology of the maxilla and mandible encom-passes the spectrum of pathology, because both systemic and unique diseases occur in these locations. Conditions previously considered 'dental' or removed from the consideration of the general surgical pathologist are being encountered with increasing frequency.

Inflammatory Diseases

The majority of inflammatory conditions of the jaws have a dental origin. Untreated dental caries eventually leads to inflammation of the pulpal or soft tissue portions of teeth that are unable to respond and heal adequately. This results in inflammation of the cancellous bone and connective tissue surrounding the dental root apices.

Dental granuloma (localized osteitis) is ordinarily detected in a dental roentgenogram. Grossly, the lesion rarely measures over 1.5 cm in diameter. Microscopically, it consists of a rounded collection of chronic inflammatory cells rich in histiocytes and surrounded by dense fibrous tissue. Degeneration can occur in the center, leading to cavity formation and the development of a radicular or periapical cyst.

Osteomyelitis of the jaws of bacterial etiology usually represents an additional consequence and extension of dental or periodontal infection. Acute, subacute, and chronic forms exist. Some of the latter are of the sclerosing (Garré's osteomyelitis) type. Hematogenous osteomyelitis is encountered more rarely, symptoms such as pain, fever, and soft tissue swelling or redness in later stages are usually present. Smooth, regular, and atrophic loss of the covering mucosa is a late finding, and the exposed bone appears dull and devitalized. Radiographic features of osteomyelitis are subtle, irregular, ill-defined, and predominantly radiolucent lesions. A sequestrum is more often identified at the time of surgical exploration than during examination of X-ray films. Acute suppurative inflammation and resorptive scalloping of margins of nonvital bone within a large portion of maxilla or mandible are the main microscopic findings. *Staphylococcus aureus* is the organism most commonly cultured. Anaerobic bacteria have also been demonstrated to be important. Tuberculosis, mucormycosis, aspergillosis, and candidiasis have also been causally identified in osteomyelitis of the jaws.

Simple Bone Cyst

Simple bone cyst usually occurs in young patients as a sharply outlined unilocular radiolucent mass. It is usually located in the body or symphyseal area of the mandible and can assume a large size. In older patients it may also involve the maxilla. It is also known as traumatic, solitary, or hemorrhagic cyst, but there is a history of trauma in only one-half of the cases, and the content of the cyst is rarely hemorrhagic. Actually, a little is observed within the cavity at surgery in the typical case; this feature is analogous to that seen in solitary bone cyst, of which simple bone cyst may be the gnathic counterpart. Morphologically, the cavity is entirely intraosseous and not lined by epithelium. Surgical samples from the periphery show instead a delicate fibrovascular lining of unremarkable appearance. A few osteoclast-like giant cells and hemosiderin-laden macrophages may be present. Surgical exploration with thorough curettage is the treatment of choice. Recurrence has been observed but is distinctly uncommon; it is said to be more frequent in the cysts having a thickened wall with dysplastic bone formation.

Giant Cell Lesions

Lesions of the jaws that feature large numbers of osteoclast-like, multinucleated giant cells include the following major entities: Central giant cell granuloma, cherubism, giant cell tumor (osteoclastoma), fibro-osseous lesions, hereditary hyperparathyroidism—jaw tumor syndrome, and aneurysmal bone cyst.

Central Giant Cell Granuloma

Central giant cell granuloma is the most common giant cell lesion and its pathogenesis is unknown. Some have suggested history of trauma could be a cause , it occurs due to the organization of slow, minute, recurrent hemorrhages, hence the alternative name reparative giant cell granuloma. This condition affects children and young adults, predominantly females, and occurs almost twice as frequently in the mandible as in the maxilla, particularly in the anterior region. It produces a cystic lesion of the bone, which microscopically shows large numbers of multinucleated giant cells, a cellular vascular stroma, and often new bone formation. The osteoclast-like giant cells have a patchy distribution, usually associated with areas of hemorrhage.

Benign Fibro-osseous Lesions

Several types of tumor and tumor-like conditions composed of benign fibro-osseous tissue exist. Their histologic features are very similar, while their clinical behavior can be very different.

Fibrous Dysplasia

Fibrous dysplasia can be polyostotic or monostotic, the microscopic appearance of the two forms being essentially the same. The polyostotic form may be accompanied by pigmented skin lesions, endocrine dysfunction presenting with precocious puberty in females, and other anomalies (Albright syndrome). Both mono-stotic fibrous dysplasia and Albright syndrome are associated with a somatic mutation of the GNAS1 gene. Fibrous dysplasia confined to jawbones is sometimes referred to as the craniofacial form of the disease. Congenital or hereditary fibrous dysplasia in siblings has been reported and should not be confused with cherubism.

Clinically, painless and sometimes dramatic swellings of the maxilla or mandible are observed that are characteristically unilateral. Young individuals are usually affected, the mean age at time of diagnosis in most series being from 25 to 35 years. The lesions tend to become static as skeletal maturity is reached. The radiographic appearance varies from cystic or radiolucent to sclerotic or radiopaque, and the margins tend to be ill-defined. The histologic appearance of fibrous dysplasia in its usual, most recognizable form is characterized by the presence of C-shaped or Chinese figure-like trabeculae of woven or immature bone within a proliferating fibroblastic stroma. Osteoblastic rimming of these trabeculae is usually absent.

Cementoma

Cementoma (periapical and focal cemental or cemento-osseous dysplasia) is a relatively common disorder, being detectable radiographically in 0.3% of the adult population. It is usually multiple and asymptomatic, is limited to small regions surroun-ding apices of teeth, and ordinarily does not require treatment. It is thought to be of periodontal ligament origin and non-neoplastic in nature. Mandibular incisor regions of female adults are usually involved. Occasionally, a single tooth is affected, and this may become a surgical specimen. Microscopically, the most typical feature is the presence of curvilinear trabeculae ('ginger root' pattern) or irregularly shaped cementum-like masses. The main differential diagnosis is with cemento-ossifying fibroma, which shows thin isolated trabeculae with prominent osteoblastic rimming.

Benign osteoblastoma can occur in the jaw, sometimes in intimate relationship to a dental root surface. The clinical course is usually innocuous, the lesion often stabilizing as a heavily calcified nodule. However, the fact that some lesions are locally aggressive indicates that surgical excision is the treatment of choice.

Microscopically, this lesion features irregular osteoid and bone formation within proliferative fibrovascular connective tissues. Plump osteoblasts are seen rimming the newly formed trabeculae. Osteoblastomas exhibiting a prominent epithelioid configuration of the osteoblasts are referred to as aggressive and are regarded by some as low-grade osteosarcomas.

Epithelial Cysts

Epithelium-lined cysts of the maxilla or mandible are among the more commonly encountered oral diseases from both the clinician's and the pathologist's perspective. Most cannot be identified specifically on the basis of their histologic appearance alone, with the exception of keratocysts and calcifying and keratinizing cysts. Therefore, integration of radiographic, surgical, and microscopic findings is necessary to reach a specific diagnosis.

Two major categories of cyst exist: Odontogenic and fissural (nonodontogenic). Odontogenic cysts arise from the odontogenic epithelium and are located within the jaw (or, rarely, in the adjacent soft tissues). Fissural (nonodontogenic) cysts are thought to arise from epithelial inclusions within soft or bony portions of the region which lack the embryologic and tooth-forming heritage of odontogenic epithelium. They occur along embryologic fissure lines. Several subtypes of these two major categories exist.

Odontogenic Cysts

1. Developmental
   Dentigerous cyst
   Eruption cyst
   Gingival cyst
   Lateral periodontal cysts
   Keratinizing odontogenic cyst
   Calcifying odontogenic cyst
   Glandular odontogenic cyst
2. Inflammatory
   Radicular cyst

Non-odontogenic Cyst

Nasoalveolar cyst
Nasopalatine cyst
Palatal cyst
Dermoid and epidermoid cyst

DEVELOPMENTAL ODONTOGENIC CYSTS

Developmental odontogenic cysts account for 10% of all cysts of the jaws. The odontogenic keratocyst and the follicular cyst account for 8%, whereas all other developmental odontogenic cysts account for the other 2% (Trimble, 1986). Emphasis will be placed on the two most common lesions in this group.

Dentigerous Cyst

This cyst has also been called a dentigerous cyst because of its association with the crown of unerupted teeth, but as other types of cysts can also be found around the crowns of unerupted teeth, the term follicular cyst is more correct because of the suspected development of the lesion from the follicle of the tooth. This cyst is most frequently identified in the mandible and is associated with the completed crown of an unerupted or impacted tooth. The cyst is thought to originate from accumulation of fluid between the reduced enamel epithelium and the completed tooth crown. Its incidence is the same in both sexes and is most common in childhood and adolescence. The growth rate may be quite rapid, with lesions growing up to 5 cm in diameter in 3 to 4 years (Livingstone, 1927).

Clinical Features

Follicular cysts may get quite large before they are diagnosed and facial swelling may be the first clinical sign. They are always associated with an unerupted or impacted tooth, most commonly the mandibular or maxillary third molar or maxillary canine.

Radiographic Features

The follicular cyst appears as a radiolucent area within the jaw and is in some way associated with an unerupted tooth crown. It is usually a well-circumscribed lesion that is unilocular and has a sclerotic bony border. There may be significant expansion of the cortical plate and displacement of tooth roots or the inferior alveolar canal. The cyst may cause displacement of the associated tooth, sometimes for quite a distance.

Histology

The follicular cyst typically has a thin connective tissue wall that is lined by a thin layer of stratified squamous epithelium within the lumen. Hyaline bodies are frequently found within the epithelial lining, as well as clefts from cholesterol crystals. Some cysts may also have mucous cells within the lining, which is of importance when considering the possibility that other lesions may develop within the wall or lumen of a follicular cyst. The lesions that may develop within the cyst arise from the actual epithelial lining or from rests of odontogenic epithelium that are in the connective tissue around the cyst. Odontogenic tumors such as the ameloblastoma frequently arise from the lining of the follicular cyst. Less common but of importance is the occurrence of epidermoid carcinoma arising from the lining of a follicular cyst, or of mucoepidermoid carcinoma arising from the mucous glands within the wall of the cyst. This is the suspected origin of most intraosseous mucoepidermoid carcinomas.

Treatment

Treatment is dependent upon the size of the lesion, but enucleation and curettage is adequate. For very large lesions, decompression to allow some decrease in size is possible but the lesion should ultimately be treated with enucleation and curettage to allow histologic evaluation of the entire lesion and to prevent recurrence.

ODONTOGENIC KERATOCYST

The odontogenic keratocyst is so named because of its characteristic biologic appearance. Clinically and radiographically it may appear as a follicular cyst associated with the crown of an unerupted tooth. It may also appear associated with the root of a tooth as a radicular cyst or by itself. When it occurs by itself, it is frequently called a primordial cyst, which is a cyst that arises where there is no apparent tooth formation associated. Virtually all primordial cysts have the histologic appearance of an odontogenic keratocyst. The odontogenic keratocyst is thought to develop from the remnants of the dental lamina, which are the rests of Seres.

Clinical Features

The odontogenic keratocyst may occur in many clinical situations. It may appear at any age but is rare below 10 years of age. The peak incidence is in the second and third decades and there is a predilection for males of 1.8 to 1. Anatomically the mandible is affected more frequently than the maxilla with 75% of the lesions occurring there (Browne, 1970). The third molar and ramus areas are the most frequently involved, with the first and second molar areas following. No clinical presentation is specific. The patient may be asymptomatic until gradual expansion is noted or until a secondary infection occurs.

Radiographic Features

The odontogenic keratocyst may be identified in a variety of anatomic locations. The majority of the lesions are present in the third molar and ramus area of the mandible. The cyst itself may have several radiologic variations. Approximately 50% of these cysts have a unilocular appearance but a multilocular appearance can occur. As already mentioned, the diagnosis of odontogenic keratocyst is a histologic one and the cyst may have several radiographic appearances such as of a follicular or radicular cyst. The lesion is slow growing and will usually be well circumscribed with a sclerotic border. Teeth may be displaced and cortical perforation may be more common than in other cystic lesions.

Histology

Specific histologic criteria exist for diagnosis of a keratocyst. These include: (1) a thin, stratified squamous epithelium that is a uniform 6 to 8 cells thick, without rete ridge formation; (2) prominent columnar or cuboidal basal cell layer with dense nuclear staining; (3) a corrugated surface layer of parakeratin or orthokeratin; and (4) a thin connective tissue wall. The lumenal material may vary from a straw-colored clear substance to a creamy white keratin-filled material. The importance of the histologic diagnosis is that an untrained pathologist may mistake the odontogenic keratocyst for a simple follicular cyst. The recurrence rate for these lesions is much higher and this misdiagnosis may lead to improper treatment.

Treatment

As mentioned previously, distinguishing the odontogenic keratocyst from other odontogenic cysts is important because of its higher
recurrence rate. Recurrence rates from 10% to 60% have been
reported. The large difference in rate of recurrence may be 14
related to inconsistencies in reporting of the data and inadequate
follow-up because these lesions can take many years to recur. In a
recent review of 426 patients, a composite recurrence rate of 34%
was seen (Williams, 1991). This is consistent with other well-
documented reports citing recurrence rates of 33% (Pindborg and
Hansen, 1963) and 44% (Toller, 1972) respectively. The high
incidence of recurrence is possible due to several factors: (1) some
lesions are multilocular, making complete removal difficult; (2)
the cyst lining is quite thin and friable, which makes it easy to
leave fragments behind during enucleation; (3) odontogenic
keratocysts have been shown to have a higher mitotic rate than
other cysts, which may make any residual epithelium more likely
to proliferate and lead to recurrence; (4) the cyst itself may have
areas of epithelial budding that are left behind during enucleation;
(5) as these lesions tend to perforate cortical bone more frequently,
cystic epithelium may be located in the soft tissue from where it is
more difficult to completely remove it; and (6) the lesion is often
clinically mistaken for more benign cysts and treated less
aggressively, only to have the diagnosis of keratocyst rendered
after treatment is complete. Treatment consists of enucleation and
curettage. If the lesion is quite large, decompression with
subsequent enucleation is advantageous. In the case of the
odontogenic keratocyst, this is particularly useful because even
after a short period of exposure to the oral cavity by temporary
decompression, the lining epithelium of the cyst undergoes a
thickening and the fibrous connective tissue thickens as well. This
makes removal easier and decreases the chance of leaving
remnants of epithelium behind. It has been shown that if the cystic
lining can be removed in one piece, the incidence of recurrence is
very small; however, if the lining is removed in fragments, the
incidence of recurrence is greater than 50% . If a wedge of tissue is
removed from the mucosa overlying the cyst, the potential source
of other lesions may be removed. Once the lesion has been
enucleated, aggressive curettage of the bony walls with rotary
instruments is recommended. Others have used chemical or
cryotherapy modalities to further remove any remaining
epithelium, but data proving that this is helpful is inadequate. If

the lesion recurs, especially if it is located in the posterior mandible or maxilla, more aggressive treatment, such as marginal resection, may be indicated.

Eruption Cyst

The eruption cyst is generally recognized as the soft tissue analogue of the follicular cyst. It is entirely within the soft tissue and does not usually produce any radiographic change. The cyst will generally undergo spontaneous rupture and resolution without any treatment. The clinical appearance is that of a smooth, tense, dark blue or purple swelling over the crown of an erupting tooth. The lesion may cause some alarm for the parent and may also be symptomatically painful. If symptomatic, a portion of the sac can be excised leading to resolution of the symptoms.

Alveolar Cyst of Infants

These small cysts are also known as dental lamina cysts of the newborn. The correct term is alveolar cyst of infants and they are small discrete white swellings located on the crest of the alveolus in newborns. These small soft-tissue cystic lesions arise from the dental lamina. They are asymptomatic, require no treatment, and will resolve spontaneously.

Gingival Cyst of Adults

The gingival cyst (called the gingival cyst of adults to distinguish it from the alveolar cyst of infants) is an uncommon soft-tissue lesion. The term is used to identify a cyst that occurs in either the attached or unattached gingival tissue. It is believed to originate in the dental lamina. It occurs at any age but is much more common in patients over the age of 40. It occurs most commonly in the cuspid-bicuspid region of the mandible. The cyst is typically asymptomatic and presents as a localized swelling in the involved area. There is usually no radiographic evidence and not tendency for recurrence after excisional biopsy, which is the treatment of choice.

Developmental Nonodontogenic Cysts

The remaining 5% of cysts within the jaws are made up of nonodontogenic cysts. Developmental nonodontogenic cysts within the jaws must arise from epithelium not associated with tooth development. In the past, several entities were described as fissural cysts because they were suspected to have arisen from tissue entrapped during fusion across various fissures during facial development. It has now been clearly shown that the only true fissural cyst is the midpalatal cyst of infants. Other so-called fissural cysts such as the globulomaxillary cyst, the median alveolar cyst, and the median mandibular cyst are most likely to be developmental or inflammatory odontogenic cysts. The other two lesions within this category are the nasopalatine duct cyst, which arises from the cystic degeneration of the vestigule bilateral oronasal ducts, and the nasolabial cyst, which is a soft-tissue cyst arising from dystopic rests of the nasolacrimal.

Nasopalatine Duct Cyst

The nasopalatine duct cyst, also known as the incisive canal cyst is formed from cystic degeneration of the oronasal ducts that connect the nasal cavity to the oral cavity during development. It is the most common nonodontogenic developmental cyst. The nasopalatine duct cyst is usually asymptomatic and is discovered on routine radiographic investigation. It may also become secondarily infected leading to rapid enlargement and pain. The cyst appears as a round to ovoid or heart-shaped radiolucency lying between the maxillary central incisors. It may be difficult to distinguish a small lesion from the nasopalatine duct itself. The nasopalatine duct cyst is lined by stratified squamous epithelium, pseudostratified ciliated columnar epithelium, cuboidal epithelium, or a combination. The cyst has a connective tissue wall that may have mucous glands, nerves, and blood vessels within it. Small cysts may just be observed with regular radiographic examination, whereas larger lesions or those that become secondarily infected should be treated with enucleation and curettage.

Midpalatal Cyst of Infants

The midpalatal cyst of infants arises from epithelium entrapped along the line of fusion of the palatal processes of the maxilla. The reason for induction of this epithelium to cyst formation is unknown. It is located at the midline of the hard palate of the maxilla. It is usually asymptomatic unless secondarily infected. It may produce a midpalatal swelling. An intraoral occlusal radiograph will often show the lesion, which is a well-circumscribed radiolucency with a sclerotic border, located in the midline of the hard palate. The histology shows stratified squamous or pseudostratified columnar epithelium. Treatment is access through a full-thickness palatal flap and enucleation and curettage. Recurrence is low.

Nasolabial Cyst

The nasolabial cyst is a soft-tissue lesion developing within the labial vestibule just below the attachment of the nasal ala in the maxilla. It has been identified incorrectly as a fissural cyst in the past and does not originate from fissular epithelium but from remnants of the nasolacrimal ducts. The clinical presentation is one of upper lip swelling or of swelling within the floor of the nose. Nearly 75% of these lesions occur in women. The cyst rarely produces a radiographic appearance. Histologically, it is a true cyst with an epithelial lining with stratified squamous, or cuboidal, or respiratory epithelium. The cyst should be treated with local excision from an intraoral approach.

Inflammatory Cysts

Inflammatory cysts make up 85% of the cysts found in the jaws (Kay and Laskin, 1985). This high frequency is the result of the prevalence of dental disease, which frequently initiates the process. Inflammatory cysts result after bacterial invasion of the dental pulp leads to a chronic low-grade infection that results in a periapical granuloma around the root of the tooth. The normally quiescent epithelial cell rests of Malassez, which are within the periodontal ligament, are activated and proliferate to surround the granuloma, leading to cyst formation. These cysts then grow by mechanisms that are not clearly defined to produce the inflammatory cyst associated with the root of the involved tooth, hence appropriately named radicular cyst. When the cyst is associated with the apex of the tooth root, it is called a periapical cyst; when it is along the side of the root, it is called a lateral periodontal cyst.

PERIAPICAL CYST

The periapical cyst is well recognized as the cystic lesion most likely encountered.

Clinical Features

The majority of these lesions are asymptomatic. The associated tooth is nonvital and may have evidence of the source of the initial offending infection such as large unrestored decay, a very large filling, or a history of pain in the tooth in the past.

Radiographic Features

The radiographic presentation is fairly consistent. It is usually a radiolucent area of variable size attached to the root apex. The radiolucency is usually rounded or oval and surrounded by a radiopaque sclerotic bony periphery.

Histology

The cyst is lined by stratified squamous epithelium. Pseudo-stratified ciliated columnar epithelium may also be seen in lesions occurring near the maxillary sinus. The thickness of the lining usually varies and it seldom exhibits keratin formation.

Treatment

Treatment requires only that the source of infection be treated. This involves endodontic therapy (root canal) of the tooth to remove the necrotic pulpal tissue or extraction of the tooth. The lesion will generally resolve after this but should be followed radiographically and enucleated if it enlarges or fails to resolve.

LATERAL INFLAMMATORY PERIODONTAL CYST

The lateral inflammatory periodontal cyst is much less common than the periapical cyst. When the radicular cyst forms around an opening between the pulp and the periodontal ligament, that is, along the lateral aspect of the tooth instead of at the apex, a lateral inflammatory periodontal cyst is produced.

Clinical Features

These lesions are clinically asymptomatic except for the associated nonvital tooth.

Radiographic features

These lesions are usually small, well-circumscribed radiolucencies associated with the lateral aspect of the tooth root. There may be signs of previous tooth injury such as dental decay, or large restoration of the tooth.

Treatment

Treatment is the same as for periapical cysts.

5

Oral Cavity and Oropharynx

The oropharyngeal region represents the upper portion of the digestive tract; in addition, the oropharynx constitutes a portion of the upper respiratory tract. The oropharynx and hypopharynx share many of the diseases of the two adjacent digestive tract organs—oral cavity and esophagus—whereas the nasopharynx shares them with the two other components of the upper respiratory tract, i.e. the nasal cavity and paranasal sinuses.

For the purposes of the topographic characterization of lesions that occur in this area, the oropharyngeal region is divided into the following regions:

1. Lip, including only the vermilion surface and comprising an upper and lower lip joined at the commissures of the mouth;
2. Floor of the mouth, a U-shaped area bounded by the lower gingiva and the oral tongue;
3. Oral tongue, defined as the portion of the tongue anterior to the circumvallate papillae;
4. Buccal mucosa, which covers the inner surface of the cheeks and lips;
5. Gingiva (alveolar ridge), the mucosa covering the mandible or maxilla from the gingivobuccal gutter to the origin of the mobile mucosa;
6. Retromolartrigone, a small triangular surface behind the third molar covering the ascending ramus of the mandible;
7. Hard palate, a semilunar area located between the upper alveolar ridge and the mucous membrane covering the palatine process of the maxillary bones;
8. Base of the tongue, bound anteriorly by the circumvallate papillae, laterally by the glossotonsillar sulci, and posteriorly by the epiglottis;

9. Tonsillar area, which includes the anterior and posterior tonsillar pillars and the tonsillar fossa;

10. Soft palate; and

11. Pharyngeal walls.

The surface epithelium of this region is of stratified squamous type throughout, with greater depth than the epithelium of the skin. It lacks hair follicles and sweat glands, but may contain scattered sebaceous glands, melanocytes, and Merkel cells. It keratinizes in the areas most exposed to mastication (gingiva, hard palate, and dorsum of tongue) but not in others. The lamina propria is composed of loose connective tissue and contains mucous and serous glands of minor salivary gland type. The oral cavity is the site of numerous diseases, both congenital and acquired, affecting a large variety of tissues and systems.

Congenital Abnormalities

Dermoid cysts are seen in the midline of the floor of the mouth. Although present at birth, they may become evident only later on when secondarily inflamed. They are lined by squamous epithelium and contain skin adnexa. Heterotopic gastric or intestinal epithelium has been reported in the tongue and floor of the mouth, sometimes resulting in cystic formations. Minute cysts of odontogenic origin are commonly seen in the alveolar and palatal mucosa of newborns and older infants; they need not be biopsied. Nodules of heterotopic nerve tissue in the palate or parapharyngeal space, mainly composed of glial elements and ependyma-lined clefts. White sponge nevus, an autosomal dominantly inherited disease, is characterized by large white plaques in the oral mucosa. Microscopically there is striking intracellular edema throughout the malpighian layer. Fordyce disease refers to the presence of normal sebaceous glands inside the oral cavity, a very common occurrence. Sometimes these glands undergo hyperplastic changes and appear as discrete nodules.

Inflammatory Diseases

Chronic inflammatory lesions of nonspecific type are produced in the oral cavity by ill-fitting dentures; ragged, sharp teeth; and poor dental hygiene. Removal of the offending agent allows the pathologic process to subside. Microscopically, a combination of hyperplastic epithelium, fibrous tissue, and inflammatory cells in varying proportions is seen. The inflammatory lesions associated with the use of dentures called inflammatory papillary hyperplasia. These lesions usually located in the palate. Lesions in which the fibrous proliferation predominates are sometimes referred to, somewhat inaccurately, as *irritation fibromas*. (Scattered stellate and multinucleated giant cells can be seen throughout the fibrous tissue, then it can be termed *giant cell fibroma*.)

Geographic Tongue

Geographic tongue is mostly seen in adults, but is also seen in children. It often occurs in association with fissured tongue. Clinically, it appears as an erythematous flat zone on the dorsum of the tongue resulting from loss of the filiform papillae. The microscopic appearance is that of a psoriasiform process; there is acanthosis with migration of neutrophils throughout the epithelium to form microabscesses near the surface, accompanied by a mild inflammatory infiltrate in the lamina propria.

Tuberculosis is a rare lesion within the oral cavity. It is usually seen on the tongue as a painful ulcer, but it also may occur on the buccal mucosa. It nearly always is associated with advanced pulmonary disease. Microscopically, there are typical tubercles.

Syphilis may produce a gumma in the tongue or palate appearing as a painless indurated mass. Microscopically, there are granulomas with giant cells, numerous plasma cells, and prominent vascular changes.

Histoplasmosis can occur anywhere in the oral cavity and can closely simulate squamous cell carcinoma on clinical examination. Indurated ulcers, nodular lesions, or verrucous masses can be present. The usual microscopic appearance is that of a granuloma, although sometimes only a nonspecific inflammatory reaction is seen. Special stains are necessary for the identification of the fungi.

Crohn disease can involve the oral cavity and pharynx, sometimes as the initial manifestation. Oral lesions develop in about 6% of patients with Crohn disease at some stage of this disorder. The most common locations are lips, gingiva, vestibular sulci, and buccal mucosa. The lesions can manifest as edema, ulcers, or in the form of a polypoidpapulous hyperplastic mucosa. Microscopically, there are edema, dilation of lymph vessels, chronic inflammation, scattered giant cells, and, rarely, noncaseating granulomas.

Sarcoidosis may affect the oral mucosa, gingiva, tongue, hard palate, and major salivary glands.

Melkersson-Rosenthal syndrome is composed of the triad of orofacial swelling, peripheral facial nerve paralysis, and plicated tongue. *Cheilitis granulomatosa* is probably an abortive variant of this syndrome, the etiology and pathogenesis of which remain obscure. Microscopically, there is a granulomatous inflammation primarily involving the stroma of the lip.

Granulomatous Inflammations

Wegener granulomatosis may manifest in the oral cavity as a red to purple hyperplastic gingiva. On microscopic examination, there are epithelioidhistiocytes, giant cells, eosinophils, pseudoepitheliomatous hyperplasia, and, in rare cases, vasculitis. Both this condition and the so-called **midline lethal granuloma**, which may present initially as a nonhealing ulcer of the hard palate.

Tongue ulceration with eosinophilia (eosinophilic ulcer; ulcerative eosinophilic granuloma, Riga-Fede disease) may mimic carcinoma clinically. Microscopically, it shows a polymorphic inflammatory infiltrate rich in eosinophils, extending into the submucosa, muscle, and minor salivary glands. The initiating event is presumably traumatic (crush injury to the tongue muscle), hence its alternative designation as traumatic (ulcerative) granuloma. Some cases have shown T-cell receptor rearrangement and CD30 immunoreactivity, but the clinical behavior so far has been benign.

Other Non-neoplastic Lesions

Leukoedema presents as a diffuse opalescent lesion of the cheek mucosa that can extend to the lips; microscopically, the main alteration is vacuolization or intracellular edema of the malpighian cells, a change of a probably degenerative nature.

Diffuse fibrous hyperplasia of the gingiva has been traditionally described as a complication of diphenylhydantoin (Dilantin) therapy, but most cases seen today are genetically inherited, idiopathic, or associated with other drugs, such as cyclosporin A. The gingival thickening can be so extreme as to necessitate surgical removal.

Oral submucosal fibrosis, as seen mainly in Indians and Pakistanis, is a reactive process characterized microscopically by subepithelial fibrosis and chronic inflammation, accompanied by hyalinization and loss of vascularity. The overlying epithelium may be either atrophic or hyperplastic and is often hyperkeratotic. The pathogenesis is unknown. The disease is thought to predispose the patient to the development of squamous cell carcinoma.

Mucocele, one of the common non-neoplastic is referred to as extravasation mucocele and represents a focus of stromal reaction to spillage of mucus from a traumatically injured minor salivary gland. It is often seen in young individuals, the lower lip being the classic location, and the microscopic pattern is that of granulation tissue surrounding one or more spaces containing mucin. Sometimes the cysts are very superficial and simulate vesicobullous diseases clinically. The second type, named retention mucocele, occurs most often in older patients and in other locations in the oral cavity, such as the floor of the mouth and the inside of the cheek. Microscopically, a mucus-filled cyst completely lined by cylindric, cuboidal, or flattened epithelial cells is seen. An anatomic variant of either extravasation or retention mucocele is known as ranula when it occurs as a blue-domed cyst in a sublingual location, and as plunging ranula when it extends into the neck above the hyoid bone.

Necrotizing sialometaplasia is a reactive condition involving minor or—less commonly—major salivary glands; its importance lies in the fact that it can be confused histologically with squamous cell or mucoepidermoid carcinoma. The disease usually presents as an ulcerating lesion of the hard palate characterized by vascular proliferation, prominent inflammatory infiltrate, and partial necrosis of salivary glands, associated with regeneration and squamous metaplasia of the adjacent ducts and acini. Cases also have been described in the nasal cavity, gingiva, lip, hypopharynx, and maxillary sinus. The morphologic changes are somewhat similar to those seen in this region after radiation therapy. The pathogenesis is probably ischemic, and some cases have been seen as a complication of vasculitis and other primary vascular disorders. The lobular configuration that these lesions exhibit on low-power examination is an important sign in the differential diagnosis with squamous cell carcinoma. The presence of calponin-positive myoepithelial cells is a supporting diagnostic feature.

Amyloidosis of the tongue is a common microscopic finding in older individuals, usually as an isolated event but sometimes as the manifestation of a systemic disease. Only in a small proportion of cases are the deposits extensive enough to result in clinically evident disease in the form of diffuse macroglossia or a localized tumor.

Tumors and Tumor-like Conditions of Surface Epithelium

Intraepithelial Squamoproliferative Lesions

It has been rightly pointed out that the lesions grouped under this generic term continue to be among the most widely discussed, reclassified, and semantically tortured conditions in the medical literature. Part of the problem resides in the fact that different clinical and pathologic terms have been introduced haphazardly over the years and that the correlations between them—although certainly present, as given below—are less than perfect. Among the clinical terms, **leukoplakia** remains the most widely used. It has been defined as a white patch or plaque, not less than 5 mm in diameter, that cannot be removed by rubbing and cannot be classified as any other diagnosable disease, and it implies nothing about the histologic appearance. It is equivalent to the term keratosis as used more often at other sites (such as larynx) and is sometimes subclassified as homogeneous, nonhomogeneous (speckled; nodular; erythroleukoplakia), crythroplakia (which is red rather than white), and proliferative verrucous leukoplakia. The most common location of leukoplakia, as defined above, is the buccal gingival gutter. The speckled type of leukoplakia is superinfected by *Candida albicans* in over 60% of the cases.

At the histopathologic level, terms such as keratosis, squamous hyperplasia and verrucous hyperplasia have been used interchangeably, the choice depending on minor architectural differences but mainly on personal preference. When dysplasia is present, this is added to the diagnosis and the changes are graded as mild, moderate, and severe. Sometimes these dysplastic changes are accompanied by a lichenoid histology (i.e. hyperkeratosis, prominent granular layer, irregular basal layer, saw-toothed rete pegs, and band-like lymphocytic infiltrate, the condition is referred to as lichenoid dysplasia.

DNA ploidy studies have shown that about one-third of 'leukoplakic' lesions are hyperploid or aneuploid, but that the relationship of this parameter with the grade of dysplasia is poor. Nucleolar organizer region (NOR) distribution counts in dysplasia have an intermediate grade between those seen in normal mucosa and in invasive carcinoma, but there is a great deal of overlap.

Overexpression of p53 has been found in only a small minority of dysplasias. In the normal or hyperplastic squamous mucosa, expression of cytokeratin 19, epidermal growth factor (EGF), and proliferating cell nuclear antigen (PCNA) are all limited to the basal cell layer, whereas in dysplasia they are often expressed also in suprabasal cells. PCNA is most potentially useful for the identification and grading of this disorder.

Carcinoma In situ

In contrast to leukoplakia, the lesions of carcinoma *in situ* and those of microinvasive carcinoma often have a red velvety component, along with that if indurations are present it almost confirms the presence of invasion. However, immunohisto-chemical stains for basement membrane components such as type IV collagen have shown thinning and discontinuity of markers in severe dysplasia/carcinoma *in situ*.

Oral Lesions and Human Papillomavirus (HPV)

The oral cavity can be the site of a variety of HPV-related lesions, some of which are microscopically and behaviorally analogous to those located in the genital tract. These include focal epithelial hyperplasia (Heck disease), verruca vulgaris, condyloma acumi-natum, and squamous papilloma. Heck disease presents clinically as a well-circumscribed, sessile, pale elevation of the buccal mucosa. Microscopically, the most prominent feature is the presence of balloon cells in the malpighian layers. This disorder is very common among Native Americans and Eskimos. The verrucae, condylomas, and papillomas often exhibit koilocytosis as a sign of cytopathic effect. Atypical nuclear changes may be present, especially in HIV-positive patients. An etiologic role for HPV has also been suggested for verrucous carcinoma and squamous cell carcinoma, including some of its precursors and variants. The benign oral lesions are statistically associated with HPV types 2, 4, 6, 11, 13, and 32, and the malignant ones with HPV types 16, 18, and 33. Among the carcinomas, those with the highest incidence of HPV detection are the poorly differentiated nonkeratinizing tumors of the tonsil seen in sexually active young individuals.

Hairy leukoplakia was originally thought to be associated with HPV but is now believed to be due to Epstein-Barr virus (EBV) lytic infection. This lesion develops in patients with HIV infection and is characteristically located along the lateral edges of the tongue. Microscopically, it shows parakeratosis, acanthosis, and intranuclear inclusions in keratinocytes, associated with ballooned or ground-glass cytoplasm. There is a high incidence of superinfection by Candida organisms.

Squamous Cell Carcinoma

Oropharyngeal carcinomas have been related mainly to tobacco and alcohol, but also to syphilis, oral sepsis, iron deficiency, oral candidiasis, and Fanconi anemia. Most cases occur in men over the age of 50, although the relative incidence among women and younger patients seems to be increasing. Some cases have been documented in children, particularly in the tongue. The location of the tumors within the oral cavity was listed as follows: lip, tongue, floor of mouth, buccal mucosa, lower gingiva, and upper gingiva and hard palate. Floor of the mouth (especially at the papilla at the Wharton duct exit), soft palate, retromolar area, and ventrolateral aspect of the mobile portion of the tongue are 'high-risk areas'. They have a common lining of thin nonkeratinized squamous epithelium, with short or absent rete ridges and a narrow lamina propria.

Microscopic Features

Intraoral squamous cell carcinomas range widely in their degree of differentiation. Those located at the base of the tongue or in the tonsil tend to be undifferentiated and solid, thereby creating diagnostic confusions with large cell malignant lymphoma. Perineurial and vascular invasion are common, especially if searched with immunohistochemical markers. The epithelium adjacent to the invasive tumor often shows dysplastic changes of various degrees, all the way to carcinoma *in situ*.

Histochemical and Immunohistochemical Features

Immunohistochemically, these tumors are invariably positive for keratin. These tumors also exhibit reactivity for involucrin and desmosome-related proteins.

Biopsy, Cytology, and Frozen Section

Dentists have the best opportunity to discover early lesions of the oral cavity. It is their responsibility to examine the oral cavity carefully and to refer patients with suspicious lesions for proper evaluation and possible biopsy. The diagnosis is usually obvious in a well-taken sample. A biopsy specimen that is often much more difficult to interpret is the one taken from an abnormal-appearing mucosa some time after irradiation therapy for an invasive squamous cell carcinoma has been completed. Under these circumstances, it is better to refrain from making a diagnosis of carcinoma unless there is definite stromal invasion, because from a cytologic standpoint it is often impossible to distinguish residual carcinoma *in situ* from radiation atypia. Generally speaking, it is better to wait a minimum of 6–8 weeks after completion of the therapy before taking a new biopsy.

The main role of frozen section in oropharyngeal squamous cell carcinoma is in the evaluation of surgical margins. A good correlation has been found between presence or closeness of the tumor at the margin and the probability of local recurrence and mortality.

Treatment

The two pillars of therapy for oropharyngeal carcinoma are surgery and radiation therapy, used either singly or in combination. For most early stage lesions, the results of irradiation and surgery are very similar, so that the final decision as to which to use often depends on factors such as functional and cosmetic results, the patient's general status, and the physician's bias. Advanced cases are treated by a combination of radiation therapy and chemotherapy.

Verrucous Carcinoma

Verrucous carcinoma (Ackerman tumor) is a variant of well-differentiated squamous cell carcinoma endowed with enough clinical, pathologic, and behavioral peculiarities to justify its being regarded as a specific tumor entity. The oral cavity is its classic location, but this lesion also has been reported in the larynx, nasal cavity, esophagus, penis, anorectal region, vulva, vagina, uterine cervix, and skin (particularly in the sole of the foot). Within the oral cavity, the most common sites are the buccal mucosa and lower gingiva. Most patients are elderly males, and there is a close connection with the use of tobacco, especially chewing or snuff dipping. Grossly, it presents as a large, fungating, soft papillary growth that tends to become infected and slowly invades contiguous structures. It may grow through the soft tissues of the cheek, penetrate into the mandible or maxilla, and invade perineurial spaces. Regional lymph node metastases are exceedingly rare, and distant metastases have not been reported.

The microscopic diagnosis of verrucous carcinoma may be difficult because of its well-differentiated character. A superficial biopsy will show only hyperkeratosis, acanthosis, and benign-appearing papillomatosis. Sections of an adequate biopsy show swollen and voluminous rete pegs that extend into the deeper tissues, where their pattern becomes quite complex. The most important differential feature with squamous cell carcinoma is the good cytologic differentiation throughout the tumor. Dr Lauren Ackerman, who first described the entity, used to express this fact by stating: 'If a lesion looks cytologically like carcinoma, it is not verrucous carcinoma.' Image analysis studies have confirmed that the cells in verrucous carcinoma are larger than those of squamous cell carcinoma or squamous papilloma.

Resection is the treatment of choice. If surgery is inadequate, the tumor will recur. Radiation therapy is not recommended, since it may alter the nature of the tumor to a highly malignant, rapidly metastasizing, poorly differentiated squamous cell carcinoma.

Tumors and Other Lesions of Minor Salivary Glands

Minor salivary glands, present in practically all compartments of the oral cavity, participate in many of the diseases affecting their major counterparts, a feature that can be exploited for diagnostic purposes.

Salivary gland choristoma presents as a gingival nodule microscopically composed of disorganized seromucinous salivary gland tissue mixed with sebaceous glands.

Adenomatoid hyperplasia is a term used for a localized hyperplastic process of minor salivary glands appearing clinically as a nodule, usually in the hard palate but occasionally in the retromolar area.

Intraoral minor salivary glands can give rise to a variety of benign and malignant tumors. The hard palate is the most common location, but similar tumors also occur in the soft palate, cheek, tonsil, floor of the mouth, tongue, lip (usually the upper), gingiva, and jaw. It is important to remember that tumors arising in the deep lobe of the parotid gland may present as primary intraoral masses. With a few exceptions, minor salivary gland tumors are morphologically analogous to those located in the major glands.

Benign mixed tumors (pleomorphic adenomas), which constitute over 75% of all parotid neoplasms, make up only about half of the salivary gland tumors of the palate. They may be overdiagnosed as malignant because of increased cellularity, nuclear atypia in the often predominant myoepithelial component (*see* under Myoepithelioma), or pseudoepitheliomatous hyperplasia of the overlying mucosa.

Adenoid cystic carcinoma, mucoepidermoid carcinoma, and polymorphous low-grade adenocarcinoma (*see* later section) comprise the large majority of intraoral malignant salivary gland tumors, in contrast to the more even distribution of tumor types seen in the parotid gland. A few cases of acinic cell carcinoma and of epithelial–myoepithelial carcinoma (to be distinguished from pure myoepithelioma, *see* below) have also been described. The prognosis of adenoid cystic carcinoma is said to be better when the tumor is located in the palate than when arising in the parotid or submaxillary gland, but this may be at least partially due to the inclusion among the palatal tumors of some cases of polymorphous low-grade adenocarcinomas. Of the salivary gland tumors located in the lip, about 80% are benign. Among the malignant types, adenoid cystic carcinoma and mucoepidermoid carcinoma are the most frequent.

Some types of salivary gland tumor occur predominantly or, in some instances, almost exclusively in the minor salivary glands of the oral cavity. They include the following:

1. Basal cell adenoma: This tumor, characterized by a canalicular pattern of growth, has a predilection for the upper lip and palate (often at the junction between the hard and soft regions), where it is sometimes confused with adenoid cystic carcinoma. As discussed, some authors like to distinguish this tumor from other basal cell adenomas and designate it as canalicular adenoma.

2. Myoepithelioma: This lesion, composed of hyaline or plasmacytoid cells, usually involves the hard palate. The differential diagnosis includes plasmacytoma, oncocytoma, and even skeletal muscle neoplasms. Despite its high cellularity and the occasional presence of atypical hyperchromatic nuclei and intravascular tumor cells, the behavior is generally benign.

3. Sialadenoma papilliferum: This is a papillary tumor of the oral cavity, usually located in the hard palate and characterized microscopically by a biphasic composition. An exophytic mass of well-differentiated squamous epithelium is seen covering a

glandular component consisting of cleft-like cystic spaces lined by cuboidal or columnar epithelium; some of these glands may contain oncocytic cells, and others may exhibit squamous metaplasia. The stroma is usually rich in plasma cells. The appearance is reminiscent of both Warthin tumor of the parotid gland and papillary syringocystadenoma of skin, both at the light and electron microscopic level.

4. Inverted ductal papilloma. This tumor has a pattern of growth similar to that of inverted papilloma of the nasal cavity. It appears clinically as a small submucosal mass in the oral cavity of adults. Microscopically, there are complex invaginations formed by well-differentiated, predominantly squamous epithelium-associated microcysts, occasional mucous cells, and a lining of columnar cells. The behavior is benign.

5. Syringoma. This neoplasm has an appearance similar to that of the homonymous skin tumor of sweat gland origin, poly-morphous low-grade adenocarcinoma. This is the currently preferred term for a low-grade malignant tumor that has also been called low-grade papillary adenocarcinoma, terminal duct carcinoma, and lobular carcinoma. Adult females are most commonly affected. The palate is the most common location. Polymorphous low-grade adenocarcinoma is the second most common type of salivary gland carcinoma in this location following adenoid cystic carcinoma. Microscopically, there is uniformity of cell type but a marked variation in architectural patterns, which is responsible for the various names that this tumor has received. Tubular, cribriform, papillary, solid, and fascicular formations may appear, with frequent combinations and transitions. The periphery of the tumor has invasive features, sometimes in an Indian-file pattern, which has led to a strained analogy with invasive lobular carcinoma of the breast. Perineurial invasion is also common.

Tumors of Odontogenic Epithelium

Odontogenic tumors represent a spectrum of lesions ranging from benign from malignant neoplasm and to dental hamartomas, all arising from odontogenic residues. Occasionally an odontogenic tumor develops from a pre-existing developmental cyst. The WHO 1992 classify odontogenic tumors into benign and malignant and with major subdivisions in each category. The subdivisions for the benign neoplasms are based on types of odontogenic tissue involved.

Ameloblastoma

Ameloblastoma is otherwise called adamantinoma, adamanto-blastoma, multilocular cyst. It is a true neoplasm of enamel organ type tissue which does not undergo differentiation to the point of enamel formation. It is described by Robinson as a benign tumor, that is, "unicentric, nonfunctional, intermittent in growth, anatomically benign and clinically persistent". The neoplasm is emerged from cells which is potentially capable of forming dental tissue. Most authors consider ameloblastoma to be of varied origin. They are:

- Cell rest of enamel organ, either remnants of dental lamina or remnants of Hertwig's epithelial root sheath, epithelial rest of mallasez.
- Epithelium of odontogenic cyst particularly dentigerous cyst and odontomas.
- Disturbances of developing enamel organ.
- Basal cells of surface epithelium of jaws.
- Heterotropic epithelium in other parts of the body, especially the pituitary gland.

Ameloblastoma occurs in all areas of jaws, but the mandible is the commonly affected area. Within the mandible molar ramus area is involved three times more common than other regions. Most of the cases are reported between 30 and 40 years. No significant sex predilection has been reported.

Radiographically ameloblastoma is described as a multilocular cyst-like lesion of the jaw and the tumor exhibits a compartmented appearance with septa of bone extending into the radiolucent tumor mass. The classic radiographic appearance of ameloblastoma is "honeycomb" or "soap bubble" appearance.

In the advanced lesion producing jaw expansion and thinning of the cortical plate may be seen.

Histopathologically six subtypes are recognized, they are follicular, acanthomatous, granular cell, basal cell, desmoplastic and plexiform.

Treatment decisions for ameloblastoma are based on the individual patient situation and the best judgment of the surgeon. Surgical plan should be influenced strongly by whether the lesion involves the mandible or maxilla. Maxillary lesions behave distinctly different from mandibular lesions. The higher cancellous bone percentage in maxilla facilitates the spread of the ameloblastoma, whereas the density of cortical plates in the mandible tends to limits the spread of neoplasm. The types of treatment that have been used include both radical and conservative surgical excision, curettage, chemical and electro-cautrey, radiation therapy or a combination of surgery and radiation.

Tumors of Melanocytes

Ephelis and **lentigo** (melanotic macules) can present as solitary lesions of the oral cavity, usually the lower lip. They are more common in females and are characterized microscopically by hyperpigmentation of the basal layer, associated in the case of lentigo with elongation of the rete ridges. The term melano-acanthoma has been used when the melanocytic proliferation extends above the basal layer and is found intimately admixed with the keratinocytes. Multiple pigmented macules of the lip are one of the components of the Peutz-Jeghers syndrome and Carney complex. The presence of pigmented patches within the oral cavity (usually located in the hard palate or gingiva) is known as melanosis.

Melanocytic nevi may involve the lips, gingiva and palate. Types of nevi are junctional, compound, intramucosal and blue nevi.

Malignant melanoma of the oral cavity is particularly common in people of Japanese and black African origin. The hard palate and gingiva are the most common locations. Both pigmented and amelanotic varieties occur. Some of the tumors have desmoplastic features, especially when occurring in the lower lip. Stains for S-100 protein should be done in any undifferentiated or spindle shaped malignant neoplasm of the oral cavity. In most instances, there is some degree of atypia in this intraepithelial component. Lymph node and distant metastases are common, and the prognosis is extremely poor.

Tumors and Tumor-like Conditions of Lymphoid Tissue

Benign nodules made of mature small lymphocytes, with or without an admixture of histiocytes, are common in the oral cavity. They may represent enlarged buccal lymph nodes or hypertrophic buccal tonsils, or may be associated with cystic glandular structures ('lymphoepithelial cysts'). The most prominent of these benign lymphoid proliferations occur in the palatine tonsils and are designated lymphoid polyps or pseudolymphomas.

Malignant lymphoma is otherwise called Hodgkin's lymphoma. It most commonly occurs in the Waldeyer ring, particularly in the palatine and lingual tonsil, but it can also develop in the gingival area, buccal mucosa, palate, or lips. Most patients are in their sixth or seventh decade, but cases have been reported in younger patients and even in children. The typical clinical presentation is that of a soft, bulky mass covered by normal or ulcerated mucosa. Microscopically, most cases are of B-lineage and follicular center cell origin, of large size and with a generally diffuse pattern of growth. It is common for these tumors to exhibit a peculiar artifact characterized by a marked elongation of nuclei. T cell lymphomas can also occur in this location, as well as anaplastic large cell lymphomas. An increasing number of AIDS-related malignant lymphomas of the oral cavity of both B and T cell type can be seen in which B cell is predominantly seen.

Plasmacytomas can occur in the soft tissues of the oral cavity. It is important to distinguish them from the more common plasma cell granulomas of reactive nature, and mucous membrane plasmacytosis. Histopathologically these disorder are composed of mature plasma cells, mixture of other inflammatory cells, and are associated with fibrosis. Immunohistochemical staining for immunoglobulin light chains may help in this differential diagnosis.

Leukemia

Leukemia is a disease characterized by a progressive over-production of white blood cells which usually appear in the circulating blood in an immature form. Leukemia is considered as true malignant neoplasm particularly since the disease is so often fatal.

Langerhans Cell Histiocytosis

Langerhans cell histiocytosis is a disease that primarily affects bone but occasionally affects other organ systems and present in a multisystemic pattern. The term histiocytosis is a collective designation for a variety of proliferative disorders of histiocytes or macrophages. It is a group of idiopathic disorders characterized by the clonal proliferations of specialized bone marrow derived, antigen presenting dentritic cells called Langerhan cells and mature eosinophils. The clinical spectrum includes on one end, an acute culminant, disseminated disease called Letterer-Siwe disease and other end called eosinophilic granuloma. The intermediate clinical form is called Hand-Schüller-Christian disease. Current theory suggest a role for environmental, infectious, immunological and genetic cause.

Hand-Schüller-Christian Disease

It is characterized by the widespread skeletal and extraskeletal lesions and a chronic clinical course usually occur at the age of 5 and also reported in adolescent and young individuals. It is more common in boys than in girls. The disease is characterized by classic triad of single or multiple areas of punched out bone destruction in the skull, unilateral or bilateral exophthalmos and diabetes insipidous with or without other manifestations of dyspituitarism such as polyurea, dwarfism or infantilism. Oral manifestations include sore mouth with or without ulcerative lesions, halitosis, gingivitis, suppuration, unpleasant taste, loose and sore teeth with precautious exfoliation of teeth and failure of healing of tooth socket following extraction.

Eosinophilic Granuloma

The term is used to describe a lesion of bone which is primarily a histiocytic proliferation with an abundance of eosinophilic leukocytes but no intracellular accumulation. This disease occurs primarily in older children and young adults, and the proportion of males to females is about two to one.

Clinically, the lesion may present no physical signs or symptoms and may found upon incidental radiographic examinations of the bones. The lesions are destructive and are well demarcated, roughly round or oval in shape. The tissue of the early lesion is soft and brown and since there is no necrosis, is not friable. Later the lesion becomes fibrous and grayish.

Other Tumor-like Conditions

Giant cell epulis (peripheral giant cell granuloma) is seen in all age groups and is more common in females. Maxilla and mandible are affected with equal frequency. A soft-to-firm mass forms in the gingiva, pushes the teeth aside, and may erode the underlying bone. Microscopically, the lesion shows numerous osteoclast-like giant cells, a cellular highly vascularized stroma, and, at times, small amounts of osteoid and bone.

Granular cell tumor can involve any portion of the oral cavity, the tongue being the most common site. The overlying epithelium often shows pseudoepitheliomatous hyperplasia. A lesion morphologically similar to granular cell tumor is seen occasionally in the gingiva of newborn infants and is called congenital epulis.

Verruciform xanthoma presents in middle-aged persons as a raised, granular, or verrucous lesion of the oral cavity, usually in the gingiva or alveolar ridge. Collections of foamy macrophages in the lamina propria are covered by a verrucous and acanthotic epithelium. The lesion is probably a reactive process rather than a true neoplasm.

Vascular Proliferations

pyogenic granuloma is most commonly seen in gingiva and lip, which appears as an elevated, dark red lesion that may or may not be ulcerated. Large masses of proliferating endothelial and perithelial cells are separated by an edematous stroma containing inflammatory cells. Characteristically, the covering epithelium makes a collarette and almost meets at the base of the lesion. The lesion may regress completely or heal as a residual fibrous mass or fibroepithelial papilloma. An identical lesion occurring during pregnancy has been referred to as granuloma gravidarum or pregnancy tumor.

Hemangioma

Benign vascular tumors are largely represented by hemangiomas and lymphangiomas. Most of these are located in the tongue, where they can result in soft cystic masses large enough to interfere with speech and mastication. Microscopically, most of these lesions have markedly dilated ('cavernous') vascular or lymphatic channels. The treatment is surgical. Tonsillar lymphangiomatous polyps present as unilateral tonsillar masses composed of dilated lymph channels covered by hyperplastic squamous epithelium, resulting in a typical polypoid configuration. Other benign or borderline vascular tumors that may present intraorally are glomus tumor, hemangio-pericytoma, epithelioid hemangioma (angiolymphoid hyperplasia with eosinophilia), and epithelioid hemangioendothelioma.

Kaposi Sarcoma

It is seen with increasing frequency in relation to HIV infection, and sometimes represents the first manifestation of the disease.

The palate is the most common site. Clinically, the lesions may appear as small, well-delineated macular lesions or as larger, infiltrative nodules. Microscopically and immunohistochemically, the features are generally similar to those of its cutaneous counterpart.

Smooth muscle tumors can also occur in the oral cavity. Most leiomyomas are located in the tongue, and many are of vascular type (angioleiomyomas). Leiomyosarcomas are more common in the cheek region. Involvement of the jawbones can occur.

Rhabdomyomas

Rhabdomyoma

The term rhabdomyoma introduced by Zenker to indicate a benign tumor showing skeletal muscle cell with varying degree of differentiation and maturity. This neoplasm consists of polygonal vaculated glycogen containing cells with fine granular deeply acidophilic cytoplasm resembling myofibril in cut section.

Etiology is unknown, however, clonal balanced translocation has been found in chromosome 15 and 17. The adult form of rhabdomyoma occurs in the middle age between 16 and 82 years old and there will be male predominance. Most frequent head and neck sites of involvements are the pharynx and the oral cavity and larynx. In the mouth the floor is most often affected. In pharyngeal lesions mostly the base of the tongue and soft palate are affected. Fetal rhabdomyoma usually occur in the newborn and young children. The most common sites are post or preauricular region, face followed by nasopharynx. Both tumor types present as a nodule or submucosal mass which can become several centimeter in size.

Treatment and prognosis—both variants of rhabdomyoma are treated by conservative surgical excision. Recurrence has been reported but is uncommon. Malignant transformation has not been reported.

Rhabdomyosarcoma

Rhabdomyosarcoma, malignant tumor of striated muscle derived from primitive mesenchyme that retain capacity for skeletal muscle differentiation. It is an uncommon tumor in the oral cavity but some lesions are reported in the tongue. There are four separate types of rhabdomyosarcoma:

- Pleomorphic
- Alveolar
- Embryonal
- Botryoid

This tumor can occur at any site but they are most commonly observed in genitourinary region and head and neck region. This neoplasm arises chiefly from orbit, inner canthus, tonsil, soft palate, mastoid, internal ear, parotid, zygoma, temporal and cervical musculature. Depending upon the site of the lesion following phenomena may be recognized which includes swelling, pain, divergence of an eye, abnormal phonation, dysphagia, cough, oral discharge or deviation of the jaw. The lesion are occasionally ulcerated and may invade underlying bone and develop distant metastasis.

Treatment and prognosis—rhabdomyosarcoma is treated by radical surgical excision followed by multiagent chemotherapy. Post-operative radiotherapy is used for those cases which cannot be completely resected.

METASTATIC TUMOR TO ORAL CAVITY

Introduction

The most deadly aspect of a cancer is its ability to spread, or metastasize. Metastasis is usually referred to as spread of a disease from one site to another. Carcinoma occurs after a single cell in a tissue is progressively genetically damaged to produce a cancer stem cell possessing a malignant phenotype. These cancer stem cells are able to undergo uncontrolled abnormal mitosis, which serves to increase the total number of cancer cells at that location. When the area of cancer cells at the originating site become clinically detectable, it is called primary tumor. Some cancer cells also acquire the ability to penetrate and infiltrate surrounding normal tissues in the local area, forming a new tumor. This process of formation of a newly formed tumor in the adjacent site is called metastasis. Tumor cells may also spread to near the primary tumor. For metastasize to occur, a cancer cell must break away from its tumor, invade either the circulatory or lymph system, which then carry it to a new location and establish itself in a new site. Most tumors and other neoplasms can metastasize, although in varying degrees.

Metastasis as known, occurs by four routes, namely (a) Spread into body cavities (b) Lymphatic spread (c) Hematogenous spread (d) Transplantation of tumor cells by surgical instruments during operation or use of needles during diagnostic procedures. Hematogenous spread is the most feared consequence of a cancer when it metastasizes. It is the favored pathway for sarcomas and carcinomas as well. Malignant cells loses cohesiveness and gets detached from primary tumor and attach to and degrade proteins that make up the surrounding extracellular matrix (ECM), which separates the tumor from adjoining tissue. By degrading these proteins, cancer cells are able to breach the ECM and escape. When tumor cells metastasize, the new tumor is called secondary or metastatic tumor, and its cells are like as those in the original tumor. Malignancies involving the bones are metastatic tumors more commonly than primary tumors. The bones most frequently with metastatic diseases are the vertebrae, ribs, pelvis and skull. In constrast to it, the occurrence of metastasis from distant primary malignancies to the jaws is considered a rare disease. These metastatic tumors are usually carcinomas rather than sarcomas, which is consistent with malignancies of epithelial origin accounting for more than 80% of all primary tumors, regardless of tumor site. Jaws are not common site of metastatic bone disease with metastases to the jaws composing less than 1% of all metastatic bone lesions. Metastatic tumors to oral region are uncommon and it occurs in oral soft tissues and jaw bones. However, they tend to involve the jaw bone more than the oral soft part. About 24% of patients the metastatic tumors in the oral cavity can be the first indication of the hidden distant primary tumor.

Age and Sex Distribution

Metastatic tumor in oral region occurs mostly in patients of age 40–70 years. A study showed an equivalent sex distribution for metastatic jaw disease, though women exhibited more metastases than men 31 to 41 years of age, and men exhibited a significantly greater incidence of metastases than women 71 to 80 years of age. This is most likely a reflection of the fact that primary breast carcinoma occurs at an early age in women, whereas prostate and lung carcinomas occurs later in life in men.

Site

Metastatic tumors to the oral region are uncommon and accounts approximately 1% of all malignant oral tumors. Recently it is said that the metastatic tumors accounts about 1 to 3 % of all malignant oral neoplasms. Metastatic tumors to oral cavity may involve jaw bones or oral soft tissues. Mandibular lesions are more common accounting about 83.5% and jaw predilection by sex where found that mandibular predilection was more prominent in females than in males. In dentulous patients, 80% of metastatic tumors to oral soft tissues occur in attached gingiva, whereas in edentulous patients, they are equally distributed between the tongue and alveolar mucosa.

In the jaws mandible is the most common site and especially posterior part of mandible. Metastatic tumors to jaws may extend to overlying soft tissues, appearing to be dental and periodontal infection. Alternatively, metastasis may occur directly in soft tissues, usually gingiva.

Pathogenesis

The red bone marrow are said to be preferred sites for metastatic tumor. The scanty vascular channels in the fatty marrow do not permit ready dissemination and growth of tumor emboli. The posterior mandible are found to be detected with remnants of hematopoitic active marrow and hence may be common site for metastatic lesions. The rich capillary network of chronically inflammed gingiva has been suggested as a mechanism that entraps malignant cells. The proliferating capillaries have a fragmented basement membrane through which tumor cells can more easily penetrate. These could be the reasons for occurrence of metastatic tumors commonly in the gingiva.

Metastases of tumors in lower part of body are usually filtered in lungs. The lung metastasis is bypassed when tumor cells take up the Batson's plexus. The Batson's plexus is a valveless vertebral plexus and this vascular system bypasses lungs and venacava. The metastatic head and neck tumors in absence of lung metastasis reveal the spread of tumor cells through Batson's plexus.

Oral Presentation

Metastatic tumors show variable presentation. Tongue and gingiva are common sites of metastatic tumors. Gingival metastatic tumors in their early stages resemble hyperplastic reactive lesions. They also show polypoidexophytic growth. In the tongue it could be a submucosal mass or may present as an ulcer.

Signs and Symptoms

In a study out of 114 cases of metastatic jaw tumors the most common symptoms were pain, paresthesia, swelling, bleeding and temporomandibular joint problems. The most common jaw symptom was pain. According to another study on these tumors, pain and pathological fractures are shown to be indicators of poor prognosis.

Common Metastasizing Tumors

In a study, most common primary tumors metastasizing to oral region are breast, lungs, male reproductive system and colorectal region. Lung cancer is most common cause of cancer death. In male subjects in a study metastasis to jaws occurred frequently from the lungs than from prostate and in female subjects occurs from breast cancer, whereas both men and women had equivalent number of metastatic lesions from colorectal region. In a review the breast and lung were most common primary sites in women and men respectively. Prostate cancers are usually uncommon metastasizing to the oral cavity. Recently studies have shown, FDG-PET scanning plays important role in locally advanced prostate cancers. According to Nishimura and colleagues, the uterus was the most common primary tumor location with the most common type of cancer being choriocarcinoma, which has high occurrence rate in the Japanese population. The common sources of metastatic tumors to oral region are breast, lung and kidney. Breast is the common primary site for metastatic tumors to the jaw bones, whereas lung is the most common source for metastasis to the oral soft tissues.

In a retrospective study of metastatic tumors of jaw in Greek population from 1989 to 2005 showed two cases originating from thyroid gland, one from esophagus and one from liver. Among these four cases three were in mandible and one in maxilla.

Radiographic Features

Radiographically, metastatic lesions are most often found with ill-defined border and usually are osteolytic (radiolucent), but they may be osteoblastic (radiopaque) or mixed radiopaque and radiolucent lesions. The radiographic appearance of lesions has been attributed to a disruption of balance between osteoclastic and osteoblastic activity that occurs during normal bone turnover.

Tumor type may affect the radiographic appearance of the lesion, prostatic carcinoma metastases are classically osteoblastic while metastatic breast or renal carcinoma may be osteolytic, osteoblastic or mixed.

Management

When cancer has metastasized, it may be treated with radio-surgery, chemotherapy, radiation therapy, biological therapy, hormone therapy, surgery or a combination of these. The choice of treatment generally depends on the type of primary cancer, the size and location of the metastasis, the patient's age and general health, and the types of treatments used previously.

6

Minor and Major Salivary Glands

The major salivary glands are the parotid, submaxillary (submandibular), and sublingual glands. The parotid gland weighs 14–28 g, the submaxillary gland weighs 7–8 g, and the sublingual gland weighs 3 g. The main duct of the parotid gland (Stensen duct) empties into the oral cavity opposite the crown of the second maxillary molar. The ducts of both the submaxillary glands (Wharton duct) and sublingual glands (Bartholin duct) open in the floor of the mouth, on each side of the frenulum of the tongue.

The parotid gland is composed of a broad superficial lobe and a smaller deep lobe, with the facial nerve running between the two lobes. Variations of this anatomy and the distribution of the facial nerve occur.

Salivary gland tissue is present in many other locations in the head and neck region, where it may give rise to inflammatory conditions, benign tumors, and malignant tumors. Its location influences, to some extent, the clinical signs and symptoms, the morphologic features, and the treatment. It is found in the lips, gingiva, floor of mouth, cheek, hard and soft palates, tongue, tonsillar areas, and oropharynx.

Microscopically, salivary glands are compound exocrine glands composed of a ductal and an acinar portion. The parotid gland is exclusively serous, the submaxillary gland is mixed with serous predominance, and the sublingual gland is mixed with mucinous predominance. The intercalated ducts and acini represent the terminal portion of the system. The reserve cells of the intercalated ducts are the source of regeneration of the acinar tissue and the terminal duct system, and are thought to be the progenitors of most salivary gland tumors. However, it has been pointed out that basal and luminal cells at all levels of the duct system and even acinar cells are capable of DNA synthesis and mitosis, and therefore they all have the potential to give rise to neoplasms.

Sialolithiasis

A stone in the salivary ducts or glands is called sialolithiasis. They are otherwise called salivary duct stone or salivary duct calculus. They are formed by deposition of calcium salt around a central nidus which may consist of altered salivary mucins, desqumated epithelial cells, bacteria, foreign bodies or product of bacterial decomposition. It is the most common cause of salivary gland obstruction, it can be complete or partial.

Chemical and Physical Features

The sialolith may be round, ovoid or elongated. It may measure just a few millimeters to more in diameter, the involved duct may contain a single stone or many stones, the surface of the calculi is rough, which may cause the duct lining to undergo squamous metaplasia. They are usually yellow and occasionally white or yellowish to brown in color. It consists mainly of calcium phosphate a smaller amount of calcium carbonates, organic materials and water. Submandibular stones tend to be larger than those of the parotid or other minor glands.

Calculi may form in the major ducts of the submaxillary, sublingual, and parotid glands, sometimes in a multicentric and bilateral fashion. They are more common in the submaxillary gland than in the parotid gland, presumably because in the former the saliva is more saturated with calcium salt and it is more long and irregular in its course. Rarely, they affect minor salivary glands. Some of the stones have a foreign body or bacterial nidus. Others do not have an identifiable nidus, are laminated, and are composed of the crystalline compound carbonate apatite. The formation of calculi blocks secretion produces swelling of the distal salivary gland tissue. If ductal obstruction persists, the gland becomes inflamed and indurated as acinar tissue is destroyed. With obstructed ducts of the submaxillary and sublingual glands, marked induration can occur in the floor of the mouth that may be mistaken for neoplasm by palpation. The duct orifices become erythematous and swollen. Radiographic examination may demonstrate a radiopaque mass, and sialography will show partial or total blockage of the duct. The stones can also be demonstrated by ultrasound. Microscopic examination of glands that have been affected by stones shows dilation of ducts, at times squamous metaplasia of the epithelium, moderate to prominent chronic inflammation, and a variable destruction of acinar tissue. Degenerative changes in the secretory and myoepithelial cells are also apparent at the immunohistochemical and ultrastructural levels.

Treatment and Prognosis

Small calculi may sometimes be removed by manipulation or increasing the salivation by sucking a lemon, leading to expulsion of the stone. An intravenous antibiotic is given for bacterial infection due to persistent obstruction of the duct. The largest stone almost always require surgical removal. Piezoelectric shock wave lithotropsy may be an alternative to surgical removal.

Sialadenitis

Sialadenitis is an insidious inflammatory disease of the major salivary gland characterized by intermittent swelling of the glands which may lead to the development of clinically obvious fibrous masses. It is most common in adults particularly males.

One of the more common causes of sialadenitis is recent surgery (especially abdominal surgery), after which an acute parotitis (surgical mumps) may arise because the patient has been kept without food or fluids (NPO) and has received atropine during the surgical procedure. Other medications that produce xerostomia side effect can also predispose patients to such an infection. Most cases of acute bacterial sialadenitis are due to *Staphylococcus aureus* but they may also arise from streptococci or other organisms. Non-infectious causes of salivary inflammation include Sjögren syndrome, sarcoidosis, radiation therapy and various allergens.

Acute sialadenitis can be localized to one salivary gland (usually parotid or submaxillary) or be the expression of a systemic infection. Viral sialadenitis (rarely seen as a surgical specimen or biopsy) can be caused by paramyxovirus (mumps), Epstein-Barr virus, coxsackievirus, and influenza A and parainfluenza viruses. Acute suppurative sialadenitis is generally caused by *Staphylococcus aureus*, Streptococcus species, and gram-negative bacteria. Dehydration, malnutrition, immunosuppression, and sialolithiasis are predisposing factors. Once an abscess has formed, surgical drainage may be necessary.

Chronic sialadenitis in the form of mild lymphocytic infiltration of the major salivary gland unaccompanied by clinical symptoms is relatively common. Some cases are of focal obstructive nature and are accompanied by various degrees of parenchymal atrophy, fibrosis, and microliths others, more common in females, are age related, have a high statistical association with rheumatoid arthritis, and are probably immune mediated. In clinically apparent cases, sialolithiasis is the most common cause.

Kuttner tumor is a chronic sclerosing sialadenitis of the sub-mandibular gland. This disorder, which is usually unilateral, is characterized by a plasmacytic and lymphocytic periductal infiltrate eventually leading to encasement of ducts in thick fibrous tissue. The lobular architecture is preserved. The lymphocytes that infiltrate the epithelial component are mainly B cells. The plasma cells contain abundant IgG4, suggesting that Kuttner tumor is part of the widening spectrum of IgG4-associated diseases. Cases in which the lymphoid infiltrate is very florid can simulate marginal zone B cell lymphoma. Surgical excision may be necessary in some cases.

Granulomatous sialadenitis can result from tuberculosis, mycosis, sarcoidosis, or duct obstruction from calculi or malignant tumors. In the latter instance, the granulomas result from rupture of ducts and may contain small pools of mucin. A xanthogranulomatous variant of sialadenitis has also been described. A fact to remember before making the clinical or pathologic diagnosis of parotitis is that the condition can be simulated by inflammatory processes involving intraparotid or periparotid lymph nodes.

Kimura disease can involve the salivary glands (especially the parotid) by spread from adjacent lymph nodes.

Benign lymphoepithelial cysts are lesions of the parotid or upper cervical lymph nodes characterized by multilocular cystic formations lined by glandular or squamous epithelium surrounded by a florid lymphoid hyperplasia with prominent germinal centers. The amount of the lymphoid component is variable. The cyst lining is often infiltrated by lymphocytes. We favor the interpretation that this is an acquired process resulting from the proliferation of branchial pouch-derived or analogous epithelium induced by the lymphoid hyperplasia, probably through a specific interaction between the epithelial cells and a subset of lymphocytes. Other examples of this phenomenon in the head and neck areas are branchial cleft cyst, the branchial cleft cyst-like formations sometimes seen in Hashimoto thyroiditis, and multilocular thymic cyst.

Mikulicz disease (benign lymphoepithelial lesion) most often presents as a slowly increasing and eventually striking enlargement of the salivary and lacrimal glands. This enlargement is usually bilateral and symmetric, but it can also be unilateral and localized, at least at the clinical level. If an infection develops, the process may subside only to recur when the infection is gone.

Sjögren syndrome is a chronic, systemic autoimmune disorder that principally involves the salivary and lacrimal glands, resulting in xerostomia (dry mouth) and xerophthalmia (dry eyes). The effects on the eye often are called keratoconjunctivitis sicca (sicca = dry), and the clinical presentation of both xerostomia and xerophthalmia is also sometimes called the sicca syndrome. Two forms of the disease are recognized:

1. Primary Sjögren syndrome (sicca syndrome alone; **no other autoimmune disorder is present**)
2. Secondary Sjögren syndrome (the patient manifests sicca **syndrome in addition to another associated autoimmune disease**)

The cause of Sjögren syndrome is unknown. Although it is not a hereditary disease per se, there is evidence of a genetic influence. Relatives of affected patients have an **increased frequency of other autoimmune diseases**. In addition, certain histocompatibility antigens (HLAs) are found with greater frequency in patients with Sjögren syndrome. HLA-DRw52 is associated with both forms of the disease; HLA-B8 and HLA-DR3 are seen with increased frequency in the primary form of the disease. It has been suggested that viruses, such as Epstein-Barr virus or human T cell lymphotropic virus, may play a pathogenetic role in Sjögren syndrome, but evidence for this is still speculative.

PLEOMORPHIC ADENOMAS

The PA is the commonest benign salivary gland tumor and the commonest salivary tumor overall, although it is comparatively rare in young children. It is slow growing and can reach giant proportions if neglected, and there is a 2–4% malignant change. PAs will recur if the tumor is inadequately removed. Although PAs have a pseudo-capsule of compressed fibrous tissue, the buds and pseudopodia from the tumor involve the capsule so that simple enucleation will leave tumor remnants and lead to multifocal recurrence. The concept of whether the capsule is incomplete and whether pseudopodia of the tumor involves the parotid tissue is currently being questioned, and with it the need for complete superficial parotidectomy. Although parotidectomy is designed to remove PAs with a cuff or margin of normal tissue to prevent recurrence, the tumor's proximity to the facial nerve frequently means that the dissection at some points leaves no tissue around the capsule. In a recent histologic analysis of the capsular form in PAs, 81% showed capsular exposure following parotidectomy or submandibular gland excision.

Treatment

Treatment of the palatal pleomorphic adenoma is based on the realization that this tumor does not possess a capsule. This notwithstanding, the tumor does exhibit a "pseudocapsule" represented by a loose fibrillar network surrounding the tumor. In addition, the periosteum on the superior aspect of the tumor does serve as a very competent anatomic barrier such that palatal bone may be preserved in this tumor surgery, even when the bone has been "cupped out" clinically and radiographically. Under such circumstances, the pleomorphic adenoma does not invade bone histologically such that bone resection is not warranted.

If the capsule of the tumor is ruptured during surgery, then recurrence is not inevitable and perhaps liberal irrigation with sterile water followed by normal saline may be tumoricidal. When recurrence occurs it is frequently multinodular and requires more radical en bloc surgery with excision of the previous scar, muscle, overlying skin, and facial nerve if they are involved.

WARTHIN'S TUMOR

This is the second commonest benign tumor of the parotid. If it is diagnosed when small and asymptomatic, it may not require treatment in an old or infirmed patient. There is a 12% incidence of multiple ipsilateral or bilateral tumors. There appears to be a link to heavy smoking and bilateral Warthin's tumors (Klussman, Wittekindt, and Preuss et al. 2006). Eight percent of these tumors occur in extra-parotid cervical lymph nodes and may be found at the time of parotidectomy or serendipidously in neck dissection specimens. Treatment is as for PA. Warthin's tumors have a tendency to occur in the parotid tail, where the majority of parotid lymph nodes occur, so partial parotidectomy is often all that is required.

Canalicular Adenoma

The canalicular adenoma is a benign tumor that has a significant predilection for the upper lip. In the past, this tumor was adenomas. The canalicular adenoma classically occurs in the upper lip in elderly women. In fact, canalicular adenomas typically affect an older population compared to pleomorphic adenomas. The canalicular adenoma is typically an asymptomatic, slow-growing, and freely moveable mass that uncommonly exceeds 2 cm in widest diameter. It may resemble mucoceles, which are uncommonly located in the upper lip. Of the 121 canalicular adenomas in the AFIP files, 89 of them occurred in the upper lip. The second most common site was the buccal mucosa. The tumor is encapsulated such that an excision of the tumor in any anatomic site in a pericapsular fashion represents a curative surgery provided that tumor spillage does not occur. The canalicular adenoma is multifocal in 20% of cases. If recurrence is believed to have occurred, it might actually represent a new primary tumor.

Mucoepidermoid Carcinoma

The mucoepidermoid carcinoma is the second most common tumor of the salivary glands overall, the most common salivary gland malignancy overall, and the most common minor salivary gland malignancy. During the greater than 60 years since its first description, this neoplasm has generated significant debate regarding the possible existence of a benign variant, the optimal number of grades, and the proper treatment for certain minor salivary gland lesions. The term "mucoepidermoid tumor" was first introduced by Stewart, Foote, and Becker in 1945.

The mucoepidermoid carcinoma is the most common salivary gland malignancy in children. Although most of these tumors are noted in the parotid gland, the palate is the second most common site of involvement. Most appear to occur in teenagers, and the majority are low-grade or intermediate-grade histology. Mucoepidermoid carcinoma in children appears to follow a more favorable course with cure rates of 98–100%.

Treatment

Surgical treatment of the mucoepidermoid carcinoma of minor salivary gland origin is primarily a function of the anatomic site of the tumor and its histologic grade. Those arising in the palate are not only the most common but also the most variable insofar as surgical treatment is concerned. It is the histologic grade that is of utmost importance when determining treatment in the palate. Large series show that low-grade cancer is most common in this anatomic site. Incisional biopsy is clearly essential to establish the histopathologic diagnosis, as previously described. Computerized tomograms are essential in planning surgical treatment of palatal mucoepidermoid carcinomas, as they assess the involvement of the underlying palatal bone. When the palatal bone does not appear to be involved by the cancer, a bone-sparing, periosteal sacrificing wide local excision with split thickness sacrifice of the soft palate musculature is the surgical treatment of choice.

Adenoid Cystic Carcinoma

Like the mucoepidermoid carcinoma, the adenoid cystic carcinoma is a very diverse tumor with three histologic variants. These have been described morphologically rather than by grade as is the case with the mucoepidermoid carcinoma, and include the tubular, cribriform, and solid variants. The adenoid cystic carcinoma is characteristically slow growing, with a high propensity for recurrent disease. It is highly infiltrative, exhibits profound neurotropism, and is associated with a dismal long-term survival rate. This malignancy was fi rst described by Theodor Billroth in 1859 and referred to as "cylindroma". In 1953 Foote and Frazell proposed the currently accepted nomenclature, adenoid cystic carcinoma. The palate was the most common site affected in the minor salivary glands, followed by the tongue. Adenoid cystic carcinoma accounts for 8.3% of all palatal salivary gland tumors and 17.7% of all malignant palatal salivary gland tumors.

Treatment

From a surgical standpoint, adenoid cystic carcinoma is probably the most challenging salivary gland tumor for the surgeon. While straightforward to perform in most cases, radical resection is fraught with recurrences and ultimate distant metastases. This not withstanding, palatal tumors should be managed with radical maxillectomy, observing 1–2 cm linear margins, and with resection of the greater palatine neurovascular bundle to foramen rotundum with frozen section guidance.

Polymorphous Low-Grade Adenocarcinoma

In 1983 two separate investigations reported on low-grade adenocarcinomas of minor salivary glands referred to as "terminal duct carcinoma" and "lobular carcinoma". Terminal duct carcinoma was suggested to specify the histogenesis of the tumor, which was thought to be the progenitor cell of the terminal duct.

High-power evaluation of polymorphous low-grade adeno-carcinoma and adenoid cystic carcinoma may permit the distinction between the two malignancies, as adenoid cystic carcinoma shows ductal type structures lined by multiple cells in thickness, while polymorphous low-grade carcinoma shows ductal-type structures more commonly lined by single cell layers. An Indian filing pattern is also seen in polymorphous low-grade adenocarcinoma. The common morphologic features of poly-morphous low-grade adenocarcinoma and adenoid cystic carcinoma have led researchers to investigate methods of distinguishing these diagnoses.

Treatment

Polymorphous low-grade adenocarcinoma requires surgery with curative intent.

The surgical procedure is based on the anatomic site. Surgical removal of these tumors in the palate requires a thorough assessment of the palatal bone with computerized tomograms. Bone involvement by this tumor is not an inherent property of this neoplasm but rather a function of chronicity of the tumor. Since these malignancies are not fast growing, many patients have long histories of their presence, such that palatal bone infiltration by the tumor may occur over time. In addition, the character-istically deeply infiltrative nature of these tumors into surrounding soft tissues, regardless of the chronicity of the tumor, is such that the soft palate typically requires full thickness sacrifice in most cases.

7

Lymph Nodes

INTRODUCTION TO LYMPHATIC SYSTEM

The body is made of a variety of cells organized as tissue and organ system. The tissue is always bathed in tissue fluid, which is made of diffusible constituents of blood and waste materials discarded by cells. A good portion of the tissue fluid returns back to cardiac circulation via venous end. The remainder is carried by lymphatics. The tissue fluid diffuses through the permeable walls of the lymphatic capillaries to become lymph.

Constituents of Lymphatic System

1. Lymph
2. Lymph vessels and capillaries
3. Lymph nodes
4. Lymphoid organs
5. Diffuse lymphoid tissue
6. Bone marrow

Types of Lymphoid Tissues

1. Primary lymphoid organs
2. Secondary lymphoid organs
3. Tertiary lymphoid organs

Lymphocytes play a vital and central role in all the lymphoid tissues and organs.

Primary Lymphoid Organs

They are areas where pre T and pre B lymphocytes mature into naïve T and B cells. The primary lymphoid organs are fetal liver, adult bone marrow and thymus. The naïve T and B cells mature in the absence of foreign antigen and leave the primary lymphoid organ.

Secondary Lymphoid Organs

They are spleen, lymph nodes, tonsils and adenoids, NALT (Nose associated lymphoid tissue), Payer's patches and MALT(mucosa associated lymphoid tissue). The secondary lymphoid organs and MALT concentrate the antigens received from local sites and also receive antigen presenting cells in efficient numbers. MALT also plays a role in immune tolerance. Exposure of naïve cells to antigens leads to activation of antigen specific lymphocytes. Thus a specific adaptive immune response is generated that offers long time protective immunity.

Tertiary Lymphoid Organs

They are ectopic accumulation of lymphoid cells that arise in non-lymphoid organs, that arise as a consequence of chronic inflammation. This causes lymphoid neogenesis or lymphoid neo-organogenesis.

Functions of Lymphatic System

1. **Tissue drainage:** Most of the tissue fluid returns via the capillaries at the venous end into main stream but about 3–4 liters fluid still remains in tissue which is drained passively by lymph vessels, failing which fluid becomes tissue logged and results in fall of blood volume.
2. **Immunity:** Lymphatic organs and nodes along with bone marrow are responsible for production and maturation of lymphocytes.
3. **Fat absorption:** This happens in the lymph vessels of the villi in the intestine which take up fat and fat-soluble materials that actually give lymph an off white or light yellow color.

Lymph Nodes

Human body is constantly confronted by numerous invading pathogens. To provide defense against these pathogens and foreign substances, a chain of well-organized and compartmentalized lymph nodes are present clustered in small groups at all strategic locations. They are the center for mechanical filtration of foreign substances in the lymph and act as site for antigen presentation, lymphocyte activation, differentiation and proliferation. Lymph nodes are present throughout the body, but more concentrated in areas draining organs and with environmental contact, as in these areas antigenic contact is constant and most often.

A young adult will have around 450 lymph nodes. Human brain is the only organ that does not depend on lymphatics but drain its extracellular fluid through CSF and the Virchow Robin spaces.

Lymph Node Anatomy

The lymph node is one of the major anatomic components of the immune system.

The three major regions of a lymph node are the *cortex*, *paracortex*, and *medulla*. The cortex is situated beneath the capsule, and represents the compartment where most lymphoid follicles reside. The medulla, close to the hilum, grows in the form of cords. It is rich in lymph sinuses, arteries, and veins but contains only a minor lymphocytic component. Both cortex and medulla represent B zones and are therefore associated with humoral types of immune response. The appearance of the follicles varies according to their state of activity. Primary follicles appear as round aggregates of lymphocytes; secondary follicles appear following antigenic stimulation and are characterized by the presence of germinal centers. The cells present in these formations are B lymphocytes known as follicular center cells (centroblasts and centrocytes or small and large cleaved and noncleaved cells), macrophages, and follicular dendritic cells. The germinal center shows polarization toward the side of antigen stimulation and is surrounded by a mantle of small B lymphocytes. Proliferated germinal centers are always indicative of humoral antibody production. Under conditions of intense antigenic stimulation, they also can appear within the medullary cords.

The paracortex is the zone situated between the cortex and the medulla, which contains the mobile pool of T lymphocytes responsible for cell-mediated immune responses. A characteristic feature is the presence of postcapillary venules, which are identifiable by their lining of high endothelial cells and the presence of lymphocytes migrating through their cytoplasm. Another cell type present in the paracortex is the interdigitating dendritic cell, a member of the accessory immune system. Expansion of the paracortex is indicative of a cell-mediated immunologic reaction. The number of lymphocytes within the lumen and wall of postcapillary venules gives a rough indication of the degree of lymphocyte recirculation.

Afferent lymph vessels penetrate the nodal capsule to open into the marginal sinus; this communicates with an intricate intranodal sinus network that merges into efferent lymph vessels exiting the node at the hilum. The endothelial lining of the outer (subcapsular) side of the marginal sinus is nonphagocytic and similar to that of the afferent and efferent vessels; the lining of the intranodal sinuses has strong phagocytic properties (littoral cells or sinus-lining histiocytes). The main arteries and veins pass through the hilum and radiate to the medulla, paracortex, and inner part of the cortex; other blood vessels penetrate the capsule to supply the superficial cortex and a small area surrounding the trabeculae.

Lymph Node Evaluation

The proper examination of a lymph node is a complicated task that may require the performance of a variety of specialized procedures depending on the nature of the case.

Biopsy

Selection of the lymph node to be biopsied is of great importance. In cases of generalized lymphadenopathy, inguinal nodes are to be avoided whenever possible because of a high frequency of nonspecific chronic inflammatory and fibrotic changes. Axillary or cervical nodes are more likely to be informative. Whenever possible, the largest lymph node in the region should be biopsied. Small superficial nodes may show only nonspecific hyperplasia, whereas a deeper node of the same group may show diagnostic features.

Adherence to a strict technique for the preparation of lymph nodes in the pathology laboratory is of paramount importance. The specimen should be received fresh in the laboratory immediately after excision, bisected as soon as it is received, and sampled for the appropriate studies. The portion to be embedded in paraffin (which should not exceed 3 mm in thickness) can be placed in 10% buffered formalin and/or a mercury-containing fixative. As a routine procedure, initial examination of a preparation stained with hematoxylin–eosin is perfectly adequate, followed by whatever additional stains and special techniques the nature of the case may be required.

A technique that complements the study of tissue sections and that is too often neglected is the examination of touch preparations from the cut surface of the fresh lymph node stained with Giemsa or Wright solution. This is particularly useful in the evaluation of lymphoma and leukemia, and in the initial triage of the specimen (such as sending tissue for culture if granulomas are seen). For instance, granulocytic leukemia can closely simulate large cell lymphoma in a hematoxylin–eosin stained section, but an imprint will readily distinguish the two conditions.

Needle Biopsy

Core needle biopsy is adequate for the diagnosis of metastatic carcinoma. Although not preferred for the evaluation of primary lymphoid disorders, core biopsies are increasingly used nowadays, putting pressure on the pathologist to render a diagnosis based on limited amounts of tissue. Compression artifact is very common in core biopsies, with the cells appearing smaller and the nuclei appearing darker compared with those seen in excisional biopsies. Very often, more extensive immunohistochemical evaluation is required to maximize the information obtainable from the biopsies.

Fine needle aspiration of lymph nodes is particularly useful for the documentation of metastatic carcinoma. It is used most often in cervical lymph nodes but also in other locations, including intra-abdominal and retroperitoneal regions.The cytologic diagnosis of malignant lymphoma can be made in 50–75% of the cases, the accuracy being greatest in the high-grade lesions. The technique has been found most useful for the selection of a representative node for biopsy, for the diagnosis of recurrent lymphoma, for staging the extent of the disease, and for monitoring treatment. Hemorrhage, necrosis, and myofibroblastic proliferation may develop along the needle tract; the latter should not be confused with Kaposi sarcoma or other neoplasms.

Bacteriologic Examination

If there is a possibility that the node contains an infectious process, an adequate sample of the biopsied lymph node must be sent directly for bacteriologic study or at least be placed in a sterile Petri dish in the refrigerator. If permanent sections show an inflammatory process, the material can then be retrieved and studied bacteriologically. For some mysterious lesions, this technically trivial step is the one most commonly forgotten.

Electron Microscopy

Ultrastructural examination of lymph nodes can be used in a few specific diseases, such as Langerhans cell histiocytosis and various metastatic tumors. Its role in the evaluation of primary lymphoid disorders is very limited since the advent of immunocytochemical and molecular genetic techniques.

Immunophenotyping

Phenotyping of lymphoid disorders has evolved into a highly complex field, as a result of the enormous cellular diversity within the immune system and the huge number (over 1000) of markers that have become available for this purpose.

Rosetting tests with coated or uncoated red blood cells and polyclonal antibodies, which were so useful for the early characterization of lymphomas, have been all but replaced by the use of monoclonal antibodies. These have received a multitude of designations, which are more dependent on the manufacturer's source than the features of the antibody. Fortunately, an internationally agreed-upon nomenclature (the CD system, which stands for *cluster designation*) has evolved, and this has allowed for better communication among the various laboratories. Over 250 CD antigens have been identified. Many of these monoclonal antibodies are now applicable to paraffin sections (Table 7.1), whereas others can be employed only in fresh cells (from suspension, cytospin preparations, or frozen section).

Table 7.1: Principal antibodies applicable on paraffin tissue sections

CD antigen and/or antibody	Predominant normal cell reactivity	Reactivity in neoplasms	Comment/caution
Leukocytes			
CD45RB Leukocyte common antigen*	B cells and most T cells, macrophages, myeloid cells	Most lymphomas and leukemias	Plasma cell neoplasms and Reed-Sternberg cells usually unreactive; some lymphoblastic

Contd.

Table 7.1: Principal antibodies applicable on paraffin tissue sections *(Contd.)*

CD antigen and/or antibody	Predominant normal cell reactivity	Reactivity in neoplasms	Comment/caution
Leukocytes			
			and anaplastic large cell lymphomas unreactive
B lymphocytes			
C20 (L26)	B cells, except plasma cells	Most B cell lymphomas; L&H cells in NLPHL; some Reed-Sternberg cells in ~20% of classic Hodgkin lymphomas; rare T cell lymphomas	May not work well in acid-decalcified tissues; plasmablastic and plasma cell neoplasms usually unreactive; some thymomas may stain
Immuno-globulin light chains	B cells and plasma cells	B cell and plasma cell neoplasms	Diffuse cytoplasmic staining for both light chains seen in macrophages, Reed-Sternberg cells, and degenerated cells (attributed to passive uptake); cytoplasmic Ig often detectable in paraffin sections; surface Ig often requires frozen tissue
CD79a	B cells, including plasma cells	Most B cell lymphomas; B cell leukemias from pre-B cell stage	CD79a is associated with antigen receptor (Ig) on B cells in a similar manner as CD3 on T cells
PAX5 (B cell specific activator protein)	B cells, except plasma cells	B cell neoplasms, including B-lymphoblastic neoplasms; L&H cells in NLPHL; Reed-Sternberg cells in classic Hodgkin	Plasma cell neoplasms are unreactive

Contd.

Table 7.1: Principal antibodies applicable on paraffin tissue sections *(Contd.)*

CD antigen and/or antibody	Predominant normal cell reactivity	Reactivity in neoplasms	Comment/caution
B lymphocytes			
		lymphoma show moderate to weak staining	
OCT2	B cells, including plasma cells	B cell neoplasms, including plasma cell and plasma-blastic neoplasms	
BOB1	B cells, including plasma cells	B cell neoplasms, including plasma cell and plasma-blastic neoplasms	Some T cell lym-phomas can be BOB1 positive
B lymphocyte differentiation stage			
CD10 (CALLA)	Precursor B cells, folli-cular center B cells; folli-cular center T helper cells; granulocytes	Many B cell and some T cell lym-phoblastic lympho-mas/leukemias; follicular lym-phoma; Burkitt lymphoma; some large B cell lym-phomas; angio-immunoblastic T cell lymphoma	Useful in separating follicular from other low-grade B cell lymphomas; expressed by subset of myeloma; reactive with a variety of nonhematolym-phoid neoplasms
BCL6	Follicular center B cells; follicular cen-ter T helper cells; rare sub-populations of T cells	Follicular lym-phoma; Burkitt lymphomas; some large B cell lym-phomas; angio-immunoblastic T cell lymphoma; anaplastic large cell lymphoma	
MUM1	Plasma cells and plasma-blasts; sub-population of BCL6 folli-	Plasma cell and plasmablastic neoplasms; lym-phoplasmacytic lymphoma;	MUM1 may be positive in nonhematolym-phoid neoplasms, such as malignant mela-noma

Contd.

Table 7.1: Principal antibodies applicable on paraffin tissue sections *(Contd.)*

CD antigen and/or antibody	*Predominant normal cell reactivity*	*Reactivity in neoplasms*	*Comment/caution*
B lymphocyte differentiation stage			
	cular center B cells; small percentage of activated T cells	diffuse large B cell lymphoma (75% of cases); other B cell lymphomas (variable); some T cell lymphomas (variable)	
CD138 (syndecan 1)	Plasma cells and plasmablasts; some immunoblasts	Plasma cell and plasmablastic neoplasms; some large B cell lymphomas	CD138 is positive in normal epithelial cells and many nonhematolymphoid neoplasms
CD23	Mantle zone B cells, subset of follicular dendritic cells	CLL/small lymphocytic lymphomas often reactive; follicular lymphoma (some cases); mediastinal large B cell lymphoma; follicular dendritic cell tumor	Low-affinity Fc receptor for IgE; upregulated by EBV infection
T and NK lymphocytes			
Cytoplasmic CD3 (detected by polyclonal or monoclonal antibody)	T cells and NK cells	Most T cell and NK cell lymphomas; exceptional cases of B cell lymphoma can be CD3+	CD3 demonstrable in paraffin sections represents cytoplasmic CD3; this is present in T cells as well as NK cells. Surface CD3, which is typically positive in T cells but negative in NK cells (and their neoplasms), requires fresh or frozen tissue for demonstration, using different antibodies (e.g. OKT3, Leu4)

Contd.

Table 7.1: Principal antibodies applicable on paraffin tissue sections *(Contd.)*

CD antigen and/or antibody	Predominant normal cell reactivity	Reactivity in neoplasms	Comment/caution
T and NK lymphocytes			
CD2	T cells, NK cells	Most T cell and NK cell lymphomas and leukemias; few myeloid leukemias	CD2 is the sheep erythrocyte receptor
CD5	T cells, weak expression by small B cell subset	Most T cell lymphomas and leukemia; chronic lymphocytic leukemia/small lymphocytic lymphoma; mantle cell lymphoma; rare subset of diffuse large B cell lymphoma	CD5-reactive B cells may be elevated in autoimmune disorders; expression of CD5 by diffuse small B cell neoplasms useful in diagnosis; CD5 typically negative in NK cells and their neoplasms; CD5 can be expressed in nonhematolymphoid neoplasms, such as thymic carcinoma
CD7	Most T cells, NK cells	Most T cell and some NK cell lymphomas and leukemias; some myeloid leukemias	Earliest expressed antigen in T cell ontogeny and one of the best T cell markers for lymphoblastic neoplasms; most commonly deleted antigen in peripheral T cell malignancy, particularly mycosis fungoides
βF1 (T cell receptor beta chain)	T cells	Many T cell lymphomas	NK cells and their neoplasms are unreactive
CD56	NK cells, minor subpopulation of T cells	NK cell lymphomas; some peripheral T cell lymphomas; some	Also reacts with neural and neuroendocrine cells and their neoplasms

Contd.

Table 7.1: Principal antibodies applicable on paraffin tissue sections *(Contd.)*

CD antigen and/or antibody	Predominant normal cell reactivity	Reactivity in neoplasms	Comment/caution
T and NK lymphocytes			
		plasma cell neoplasms	
CD43	T cells, macrophages, Langerhans cells, myeloid cells, minor subset of B cells	Most T cell lymphomas; some B cell lymphomas; myeloid leukemias; histiocytic neoplasms; Langerhans cell histiocytosis; some plasma cell neoplasms	Can be exploited for diagnosis of small B cell lymphoma/leukemia
CD45RO	T cells, some macrophages, myeloid cells	Most T cell lymphomas, few B cell lymphomas; myeloid leukemias; histiocytic neoplasms	
T or NK cell subset or differentiation stage			
CD57	Some NK cells; subset of germinal center T cells	T cell large granular lymphocyte leukemia; rare cases of T lymphoblastic neoplasm	CD57+ cells often rosette around L&H cells in NLPHL
CD4	Most helper/inducer T cells, many macrophages, many dendritic cells	Many peripheral T cell lymphomas; histiocytic neoplasms; Langerhans cell histiocytosis	HIV receptor generally predominates
CD8	Most cytotoxic/suppressor T cells, subset of NK cells, splenic sinus lining cells	Minority of peripheral T cell lymphomas	

Contd.

Table 7.1: Principal antibodies applicable on paraffin tissue sections *(Contd.)*

CD antigen and/or antibody	Predominant normal cell reactivity	Reactivity in neoplasms	Comment/caution
Precursor cell marker			
Terminal deoxynucleoti- dyl transferase (TdT)	Precursor cells in marrow, cortical thymo- cytes	Most lymphoblas- tic lymphomas and leukemias of a T or B lineage; some myeloid leukemias	Useful as marker of precursor cell lym- phomas/leukemia
Hodgkin lymphoma-associated			
CD30	Some acti- vated B and T cells, some plasma cells	Reed-Sternberg cells in most cases of classic Hodgkin lym- phoma; anaplastic large cell lym- phomas; some B and T cell lymphomas	Embryonal carcinomas and few other non- hematolymphoid neoplasms reactive
CD15 (Leu-M1)	Granulocytes, some macro- phages	Reed-Sternberg cells in most cases of classic Hodgkin lymphoma; large cells in some B and T cell lym- phomas; histio- cytic neoplasms; some myeloid leukemias	Many carcinomas reactive; CMV-infected cells reactive; antibody of IgM isotype and thus may benefit from iso- type specific detection; L&H cells usually unreactive
Accessory cells			
CD68	Macrophages and mono- cytes; myeloid cells positive with KP1 but not PGM1 antibody	True histiocytic neoplasms; mono- cyticleukemias; myeloid leukemias positive with KP1	Reactive in granular cell tumors, some melanomas, malignant fibrous histiocytomas, and renal cell carci- nomas
CD163	Macrophages except those	Histiocytic neo- plasms; acute	Dendritic cells and their tumors are

Contd.

Table 7.1: Principal antibodies applicable on paraffin tissue sections *(Contd.)*

CD antigen and/or antibody	Predominant normal cell reactivity	Reactivity in neoplasms	Comment/caution
Accessory cells			
	of germinal centers and splenic white pulp	monocytic leuke-mia	unreactive
Lysozyme	Macrophages, myeloid cells	Histiocytic neo-plasms; many myeloid leukemias	Reactive with many nonhematolymphoid neoplasms
S-100 protein	Langerhans cells, inter-digitating (IDRC) and sometimes follicular dendritic cells	Langerhans cell histiocytosis; IDRC tumors; rare T cell lymphomas; histiocytic neo-plasms; Rosai-Dorfman disease	Reactive with many nonhematolymphoid neoplasms
CD1a	Cortical thy-mocytes, Langerhans cells	Some T lympho-blastic lympho-mas/leukemias; Langerhans cell histiocytosis	
CD207 (langerin)	Langerhans cells	Langerhans cell histiocytosis	
CD21	Mantle and marginal zone B cells, folli-cular dendritic cells	Some B cell lym-phomas; follicular dendritic cell tumors	C3d (CR2) complement receptor; receptor for EBV
CD35	Mantle and marginal zone B cells, folli-cular dendritic cells, some macrophages	Some B cell lym-phomas; follicular dendritic cell tumors; some myeloid leukemias	C3b (CR1) complement receptor
Miscellaneous			
BCL2	Nongerminal center B cells, most T cells,	Overexpressed in most follicular lymphomas and	Most useful in differ-entiating follicular lymphoma from

Contd.

Table 7.1: Principal antibodies applicable on paraffin tissue sections *(Contd.)*

CD antigen and/or antibody	Predominant normal cell reactivity	Reactivity in neoplasms	Comment/caution
Miscellaneous			
	plasma cells	some diffuse large B cell lymphomas; also expressed in many other lymphomas and leukemias	reactive follicular hyperplasia
Cyclin D1	Some histiocytes; normal lymphoid cells are negative	Mantle cell lymphoma; rare cases of diffuse large B cell lymphoma; some plasma cell neoplasms; some cases of hairy cell leukemia	Cyclin D1 is expressed in many nonhematolymphoid neoplasms
Anaplastic lymphoma kinase (ALK)	None	ALK+ anaplastic large cell lymphoma; ALK+ large B cell lymphoma; ALK+ histiocytosis	ALK also positive in some cases of inflammatory myofibroblastic tumor
Myeloperoxidase	Myeloid cells	Myeloid leukemias	Most sensitive and specific marker for myeloid neoplasms

Modified from Warnke RA, Weiss LM, Chan JKC, Cleary ML, Dorfman RF. Tumors of the lymph nodes and spleen. Atlas of tumor pathology, series 3, fascicle 14. Washington, DC, 1995, Armed Forces Institute of Pathology.

* CMV, cytomegalovirus; CLL, chronic lymphocytic leukemia; EBV, Epstein-Barr virus; NLPHL, nodular lymphocyte predominant Hodgkin lymphoma.

Immunophenotyping can be performed by flow cytometry (requiring fresh tissue) or on paraffin-embedded materials. Two major advantages of the former are rapid availability of results, and excellent assessment of surface immunoglobulin and hence B cell clonality. The disadvantages are the need for immediate handling of fresh tissue, and suboptimal architectural–morphologic correlation.

Gene rearrangement analysis

Antigen receptor genes code for immunoglobulin and T cell receptor protein molecules. B cells express immunoglobulins in both a membrane and soluble form, whereas T cells express T cell receptors, which are membrane-bound molecules. These two kinds of molecules have significant functional and structural similarities and are involved in the specific recognition of antigens by lymphocytes.

Both molecules are multi-subunit glycoproteins. Each subunit can be divided roughly into two parts: a constant region and a variable region. Variable regions of two subunits collaborate to form highly specific antigen-binding sites. A given lymphocyte, throughout its lifetime, can express only one type of variable region for each of two (or in the case of T cells, at most three) antigen receptor subunits.

Genetic rearrangements that occur within the genes of these subunits determine which variable region is expressed for a given subunit. During the lifetime of a lymphocyte, rearrangement generally occurs only once per allele or twice for a given gene, as there are two alleles for each gene. The rearrangement can be detected by Southern blot or polymerase chain reaction (PCR).

Three general types of application of gene rearrangements to the diagnosis of lymphoid neoplasms exist:

1. For the differential diagnosis between benign and malignant lesions
2. As markers for B or T cell derivation
3. As markers for the presence of multiple lymphocytic clones in a single patient (Table 7.2)

Mature B cell lymphomas almost always show clonal rearrangements of the immunoglobulin genes, although rare cases may show simultaneous rearrangements of T cell receptor genes. Mature T cell lymphomas almost always show clonal rearrangements of the T cell receptor genes, but rare cases may show simultaneous rearrangements of the immunoglobulin genes, an occurrence which is particularly common in angioimmunoblastic T cell lymphomas (20–30%), probably due to the presence of supervening Epstein-Barr virus (EBV)-associated B cell proliferation. However, precursor lymphoblastic lymphomas frequently show cross-lineage antigen receptor gene rearrangements.

Table 7.2: Commonly encountered gene rearrangement patterns and their interpretation

Antigen receptor gene status					
IgH	*Ig*	*Ig*	*TCRβ*	*TCR*	*Most probable interpretation*
R	R	G	G	G	B cell neoplasms
R	R	R	G	G	B cell neoplasms
G	G	G	R	R	T cell neoplasm
R	G	G	R	R	T cell neoplasm
G	G	G	G	G	No molecular support for lymphoma

From Warnke RA, Weiss LM, Chan JKC, Cleary ML, Dorfman RF. Tumors of the lymph nodes and spleen. Atlas of tumor pathology, series 3, fascicle 14. Washington, DC, 1995, Armed Forces Institute of Pathology.

G, germline band; R, rearranged band.

Analysis of the immunoglobulin and T cell receptor gene status in lymphoid proliferations may help in determining clonality, which generally but not invariably indicates a neoplastic process, and in determining lineage, with the caveats of possible cross-lineage gene rearrangements. Demonstration of clonal immunoglobulin or T cell receptor gene rearrangements is most commonly achieved by PCR, which has superseded the much more laborious and demanding Southern blot technique. Although PCR is a highly sensitive technique, being able to demonstrate even minor clonal populations, there can be significant false-negative results due to imperfect annealing of the consensus primers with the target DNA sequences. However, false-negative results can be significantly reduced by using multiple primer pairs against the antigen receptor gene target, such as using the BIO-MED2 primers.

Cytogenetics and Molecular Genetics

Chromosomal translocation

Several nonrandom chromosomal translocations have been detected in malignant lymphoma (Table 7.3). Remarkably, most of these translocations are associated with specific lymphoma subtypes even if exceptions occur.

Chromosomal translocation results in fusion of two separate genes, which has one of the following two consequences.

1. Juxtaposition of the regulatory elements of a highly expressed gene in the cell type (e.g. immunoglobulin gene in a B cell)

Table 7.3: Recurrent chromosomal abnormalities in lymphomas

Chromosomal abnormality	Most frequent types of lymphoma	Antigen receptor gene	Oncogene
t(8;14)(q24;q32)	Burkitt lymphoma, and	IGH	CMYC
t(2;8)(2p12;q24)	rarely diffuse large B cell	IG	CMYC
t(8;22)(q24;q11)	lymphoma	IG	CMYC
t(14;18)(q32;q21)	Follicular lymphoma; subset of diffuse large B cell lymphomas	IGH	BCL2
t(11;14)(q13;q32)	Mantle cell lymphoma	IGH	CCND1 (cyclin D1)
t(3;v)(q27;v)a	Large B cell lymphoma; small subset of follicular lymphomas	IGH, IG, IG, others	BCL6
t(14;v)(q11;v)	T lymphoblastic lymphoma; adult T cell leukemia/ lymphoma	TCR^a/TCR	Several
t(7;v)(q35;v)	T lymphoblastic lymphoma	TCRβ	Several
t(2;5)(p23;q35)	Anaplastic large cell lymphoma, ALK+	NA	NPM–ALK fusion gene
t(11;18)(q21;q21)		NA	API2–MALT1 fusion gene
t(14;18)(q32;q21)	Extranodal marginal zone lymphoma of mucosa-associated lymphoid tissue	IGH	MALT1
t(3;14)(p14.1;q32)		IGH	FOXP1
t(1;14)(p22;q32)		IGH	BCL10

Modified from Warnke RA, Weiss LM, Chan JKC, Cleary ML, Dorfman RF. Tumors of the lymph nodes and spleen. Atlas of tumor pathology, series 3, fascicle 14. Washington, DC, 1995, Armed Forces Institute of Pathology.

[a] Variable. NA, not applicable.

with the coding sequences of a partner gene results in overexpression of the latter, causing increased production of a structurally normal protein; for example, BCL2 protein as a result of t(14;18) causing fusion of IGH with BCL2.

2. Juxtaposition of the coding sequences of the two involved genes results in gene fusions that code for a novel chimeric protein; for example, t(2;5) leads to production of a protein which is partly encoded by ALK and partly encoded by NPM.

Chromosomal translocations can be detected by conventional cytogenetics, Southern blot analysis, reverse transcriptase PCR (RT-PCR) and fluorescent *in situ* hybridization (FISH). Each of these techniques has its own advantages and limitations. However, the FISH technique, either using breakapart probe or dual-fusion probe, generally offers the highest sensitivity.

Chromosome copy change and chromosomal gain or deletion

Increase in copies of entire chromosomes is common in certain lymphoma types, such as trisomy 3 or trisomy 18 in extranodal marginal zone lymphoma, and trisomy 12 in chronic lymphocytic leukemia/small lymphocytic lymphoma. Lymphomas can also exhibit deletions or gains of specific regions of chromosome, such as 6q21–25 in extranodal NK/T cell lymphoma, del 6q23.3 in marginal zone lymphoma, and gain of 3q26 in mantle cell lymphoma. These chromosomal changes can be demonstrated by conventional cytogenetics, FISH or single nucleotide polymorphisms (SNP) microarrays.

Gene mutation, amplification, and hypermethylation

Point mutations in specific genes are characteristic of some lymphoma types, including activating mutations of proto-oncogenes, such as point mutations in genes involved in regulation of the nuclear factor kappa B in some cases of diffuse large B cell lymphoma, and inactivating mutations of tumor suppressor genes, such as *A20* in various lymphoma types. An inactivating mutation in a tumor suppressor gene is often accompanied by chromosomal/gene deletion in the remaining allele, resulting in complete loss of function of the gene. Tumor suppressors genes are alternatively inactivated in some lymphomas through hypermethylation of the gene promoters, such as p16 in mantle cell lymphoma. Gene amplifications are found in some lymphomas, such as *REL* in diffuse large B cell lymphoma.

DNA ploidy studies

Examination of DNA ploidy by flow cytometry of cell suspensions from fluids or material from fine needle aspiration or from tissue sections has shown a good correlation with the microscopic grades of malignant lymphoma. Whether it provides prognostic information above and beyond that obtainable from conventional morphology and immunophenotyping of the tumors remains controversial.

Gene expression profiling

Some highly publicized studies have been published on the use of molecular profiling with the microarray technology to segregate diffuse large B cell lymphomas into subtypes and to predict survival after chemotherapy. Although microarray-based gene expression profiling has provided tremendous information on various lymphoma types, this technology has not yet been reproducibly applied in the diagnostic setting.

Primary Immunodeficiencies

The many varieties of primary immunodeficiencies can be broadly divided in three major categories according to the type of the immunologic deficit: *humoral, cell-mediated,* and *due to defects in phagocytes and other cells of the accessory immune system.* The diagnosis of these disorders is based on a variety of laboratory tests, including qualitative and quantitative immunoglobulin determinations, delayed-type skin reactions, and *in vitro* stimulation of lymphocytes. Sometimes lymph nodes are biopsied to assess the amount and composition of the lymphoid tissue. In immune diseases of the humoral type, cortical reactive centers and medullary plasma cells are scanty or absent. In diseases of cell-mediated immunity, the thickness of the paracortical area is greatly diminished. When both humoral and cell-mediated types of immunity are defective, the lymphocyte and plasma cell content of the node is practically nil, the lymph node being reduced to a mass of connective tissue and blood vessels.

Patterns of Hyperplasia

The various components of the lymph node react to various known and unknown stimuli by undergoing reactive changes, some being the expression of an inflammatory reaction and some being indicative of an immune response. The two are often present together. A similar microscopic picture may result from a variety of causes, but some agents produce a characteristic microscopic picture. When the hyperplastic change is very intense, the differential diagnosis with malignant lymphoma may become difficult and may require the application of immunohistochemical and molecular genetic methods.

Although most lymph node reactions involve several compartments, it is useful to evaluate these compartments individually, not only because their presence and relative intensity correlate with various specific disorders (thus providing important etiologic clues), but also because each of them raises differential diagnostic problems with different types of malignant processes. From a topographic and functional standpoint, the major patterns of reactive lymphoid proliferations are *follicular/nodular, interfollicular/ paracortical, diffuse, sinusal,* and *mixed.* These patterns also apply to the various types of malignant lymphoma.

Follicular Hyperplasia

The criteria laid down in the classic article by Rappaport et al and further elaborated by Nathwani et al remain extremely useful and reliable to distinguish reactive follicular hyperplasia from follicular lymphoma. In general, reactive follicles vary considerably in size and shape; their margins are sharply defined and surrounded by a mantle of small lymphocytes often arranged circumferentially with an onion-skin pattern and sometimes concentrating on one pole of the follicle (corresponding to the side of the antigenic stimulation); the follicles are composed of an admixture of small and large lymphoid cells with irregular (elongated and cleaved) nuclei; mitoses are numerous; and phagocytosis of nuclear debris by histiocytes is prominent, resulting in a starry sky pattern. The lymphoid tissue present between the follicles is distinctly different from that of the follicles themselves (although this also may be true for follicular lymphoma); it is composed of a mixture of small lymphocytes, large lymphoid cells, prominent postcapillary venules, and sometimes a prominent component of mature plasma cells.

Follicular hyperplasia can accompany a large number of inflammatory and noninfectious conditions. When the reactive follicles are particularly large ('giant'), infection by Epstein-Barr virus should be suspected. It should be kept in mind that follicular hyperplasia may coexist in the same node with follicular lymphoma or other types of malignant lymphoma.

Progressively and Regressively Transformed Germinal Centers

Progressively transformed germinal centers are the morphologic expression of a distinct type of follicular hyperplasia. They usually are seen in conjunction with more typical reactive germinal centers and are often located more centrally within the node. They are large and contain numerous small lymphocytes, the borders are indistinct, and the interphase between the germinal center and the cuff of small lymphocytes is blurred. However, residual starry sky macrophages are present, together with scattered large

Table 7.4: Differential diagnosis based upon recognition of predominant pattern in lymph node at low magnification

Follicular/nodular	Interfollicular/paracortical	Diffuse	Sinus	Mixed/other
Non-neoplastic				
Reactive follicular hyperplasia	Immunoblastic proliferations	Immunoblastic proliferations	Sinus hyperplasia	Mixed hyperplasia
Explosive follicular hyperplasia (HIV)	Viral lymphadenitis (EBV, CMV, herpes)	Viral lymphadenitis (EBV, CMV, herpes)	Rosai–Dorfman disease	Dermatopathic lymphadenopathy
Progressive transformation of germinal centers	Post-vaccination lymphadenitis	Post-vaccination lymphadenitis	Lymphangiogram effect	Toxoplasmosis
Castleman disease	Drug sensitivity, e.g. diphenyl-hydantoin (Dilantin)	Drug sensitivity, e.g. diphenylhydantoin	Whipple disease	Cat-scratch disease
Rheumatoid lymphadenopathy			Vascular transformation of sinuses	Systemic lupus erythematosus
Luetic lymphadenitis			Hemophagocytic syndrome	Kawasaki disease
Kimura disease				Kikuchi lymphadenitis
				Granulomatous lymphadenitis
				Inflammatory pseudo-tumor
Uncertain if neoplastic				
	Angioimmunoblastic lymphadenopathy		Langerhans cell histiocytosis	Systemic Castleman disease
Neoplastic				
Nodular lymphocyte predominant HD	Interfollicular HD	Mixed cellularity HD	Large cell lymphoma with sinusoidal pattern	Marginal zone lymphoma
Nodular sclerosis	Peripheral T-cell lymphoma	Small cell B/T lymphoma/leukemia		
	Mixed cellularity HD			

Contd.

Table 7.4: Differential diagnosis based upon recognition of predominant pattern in lymph node at low magnification *(Contd.)*

Follicular/nodular Neoplastic	Interfollicular/paracortical	Diffuse	Sinus	Mixed/other
HD	Small cell B/T lymphoma/ leukemia	Large cell B/T lymphoma	Mastocytosis	Nonlymphoid leukemia
Follicular lymphoma	Burkitt lymphoma	Lymphoblastic lymphoma/ leukemia	Nonlymphoid leukemia	Histiocytic neoplasms
Mantle cell lymphoma	Plasmacytoma	Burkitt lymphoma	Histiocytic neoplasms	Nonhemato- lymphoid neo- plasms
Marginal zone lymphoma	Nonlymphoid leukemia	Plasmacytoma	Nonhemato- lymphoid neo- plasms	
CLL/SLL with proliferation centers	Mastocytosis	Anaplastic large cell lymphoma		
	Histiocytic neoplasms	Nonlymphoid leukemia		
	Nonhematolymphoid neoplasms	Mastocytosis		
		Histiocytic neoplasms		
		Nonhematolymphoid neoplasms		

Modified from Warnke RA, Weiss LM, Chan JKC, Cleary ML, Dorfman RF. Tumors of the lymph nodes and spleen. Atlas of tumor pathology, series 3, fascicle 14. Washington, DC, 1995, Armed Forces Institute of Pathology.

CLL, chronic lymphocytic leukemia; CMV, cytomegalovirus; EBV, Epstein-Barr virus; HD, Hodgkin disease; SLL, small lymphocytic lymphoma.

Table 7.5: Architectural and cytologic features of follicular lymphoma and of reactive follicular hyperplasia as described in a classic and still very pertinent article on the subject

Follicular lymphoma	*Reactive follicular hyperplasia*
Architectural features	
Complete effacement of normal architecture	Preservation of nodal architecture
Even distribution of follicles throughout cortex and medulla	Follicles more prominent in cortical portion of lymph node
Slight or moderate variations in size and shape of follicles	Marked variations in size and shape of follicles with presence of elongated, angulated, and dumbbell-shaped forms
Fading of follicles	Sharply demarcated reaction centers
Massive infiltration of capsule and pericapsular fat with or without formation of neoplastic follicles outside capsule	No, or only moderate, infiltration of capsule and pericapsular fat tissue with inflammatory cells that may be arranged in perivascular focal aggregates (when associated with lymphadenitis)
Condensation of reticulin fibers at periphery of follicles	Little or no alteration of reticular framework
Cytologic features	
Follicles composed of neoplastic cells exhibiting cellular pleomorphism with nuclear irregularities	Centers of follicles (reaction centers) composed of lymphoid cells, histiocytes, and 'reticulum cells', with a few or no cellular and nuclear irregularities
Lack of phagocytosis	Active phagocytosis in reaction centers
Relative paucity of mitotic figures usually without significant difference in their number inside and outside the follicles; occurrence of atypical mitoses	Moderate to pronounced mitotic activity in reaction centers; rare or no mitoses outside reaction centers; no atypical mitoses
Similarity of cell type inside and outside follicles	Infiltration of tissue between reaction centers with inflammatory cells (when associated with lymphadenitis)

Slightly modified from Rappaport H, Winter WJ, Hicks EB. Follicular lymphoma. A reevaluation of its position in the scheme of malignant lymphoma, based on a survey of 253 cases. Cancer 1956, 9: 792–821.

lymphoid cells (cleaved and noncleaved) and occasional collections of epithelioid cells at the periphery. There is an increased network of follicular dendritic cells, a larger number of mantle zone lymphocytes, and a relatively large number of T lymphocytes. Evaluation of these features should allow the differential diagnosis between progressively transformed germinal centers and follicular lymphoma to be made with ease in most instances; however, cases exist in which this is extremely difficult on the basis of routinely stained sections.

Progressively transformed germinal centers can occur as an isolated self-limited reactive process, particularly in young men. However, they also show an interesting and still poorly understood relation with nodular lymphocyte predominant Hodgkin lymphoma (NLPHL), which may manifest itself in three ways: they may precede the development of NLPHL, they may accompany NLPHL in involved nodes, or they may appear in the absence of NLPHL in recurrent post-therapy adenopathy done for the latter. Indeed, the main differential diagnosis of progressively transformed germinal centers is with NLPHL, which should be suspected if T cell rosettes are prominent. A thorough search for the atypical cells seen in this condition should then be undertaken.

Regressively transformed germinal centers are small, practically devoid of lymphoid cells, and composed of follicular dendritic cells, vascular endothelial cells, and hyalinized periodic acid–Schiff (PAS)-positive intercellular material. These abnormal centers have an onion-skin appearance in low-power examination. Regressively transformed germinal centers are particularly prominent and numerous in Castleman disease. A peculiar form of regressive germinal centers with 'follicular dendritic cells only' has been described in organ transplant recipients.

Mantle/Marginal Zone Hyperplasia

This pattern of hyperplasia, which blends with the lymphoid subtype of hyaline vascular Castleman disease is characterized by a monomorphic proliferation of small lymphoid cells with round nuclei and clear cytoplasm which may be arranged in a nodular, inverse follicular, and/or marginal zone pattern. The main differential diagnosis is with mantle cell lymphoma. Features in favor of benignancy at the hematoxylin–eosin level are the lack of pericapsular infiltration, preservation of sinuses, scattered reactive follicles, and paracortical nodular hyperplasia. Immunoglobulin gene rearrangement studies may be necessary to settle the issue.

Paracortical Hyperplasia

Expansion of the paracortical (interfollicular) region can be nodular or diffuse. The nodular form is characteristic of dermatopathic lymphadenitis and of nodal reactions to malignancy. The diffuse form is a feature of viral lymphadenitis, drug reactions and immunoblastic proliferations in general.

Sinus Hyperplasia

The sinuses appear dilated and prominent in various disorders. The most common and least significant is *sinus hyperplasia* seen in nodes draining infectious or neoplastic processes and characterized by an increased number of macrophages in the lumen. Other reactive disorders involving primarily the sinuses are Rosai–Dorfman disease (RDD), Langerhans cell histiocytosis, Whipple disease, vascular transformation of sinuses, and virus-associated hemophagocytic syndrome.

Granulomatous Inflammation

There are a large number of diseases that can result in granulomatous formation in lymph nodes. They include various types of infection, foreign body reactions, aberrant immune reactions, and secondary responses in lymph nodes draining carcinoma or in patients with Hodgkin lymphoma and other lymphomas, whether the node is involved by the malignancy or not. Sometimes the appearance of the granulomas is such that a specific diagnosis can be strongly suggested on the basis of the hematoxylin–eosin stained slide. Features of importance in this regard are the presence and type of necrosis; number, and size of Langhans giant cells; size, shape, and distribution of the granulomas; and type of associated changes in the intervening tissue. In most cases, however, a combination of clinical, morphologic, and bacteriologic data is necessary to determine the etiology of the granulomas. It is therefore important that any node suspected of harboring a granulomatous process be sampled for bacteriologic analysis in addition to being subjected to the standard microscopic examination.

Other Cell Types Involved in Nodal Hyperplasia

Monocytoid B Cells

Monocytoid B cell hyperplasia is characterized by the filling of the sinuses by small lymphoid cells with round or angulated nuclei and clear cytoplasm, sometimes admixed with neutrophils. A variant characterized by the presence of a larger cell component has also been recognized. It was originally described as *immature sinus histiocytosis*, but marker studies have shown that these monocytoid clear cells are of B cell type. This alteration occurs most frequently in toxoplasmosis, but it has also been seen in many other reactive disorders, including cat-scratch disease, infectious mononucleosis, AIDS, and autoimmune disorders; it may also accompany malignant lymphomas, including Hodgkin lymphoma. It should be distinguished from other nodal lesions featuring cells with clear cytoplasm (such as peripheral T cell lymphomas, hairy cell leukemia, and mastocytosis) and also from a type of malignant lymphoma composed of cells with features of monocytoid B cells (nodal marginal zone B cell lymphoma).

Plasmacytoid Dendritic Cells

Clusters of cells with plasmacytoid cytoplasm, fine nuclear chromatin pattern, and small nucleoli are sometimes seen in a variety of reactive nodal lesions. Pyknosis and starry-sky pattern may be present. These cells were originally interpreted as T-associated plasma cells and later as a subtype of T cells, but then as macrophages/monocytes (plasmacytoid monocytes), and more recently as a special form of dendritic cells. They are particularly common in Kikuchi necrotizing lymphadenitis and Castleman disease, but they can also be seen in other lymphadenitis. A variety of malignant lymphoma composed of plasmacytoid dendritic cells has also been described.

Polykaryocytes

The term *polykaryocyte* is used for a type of multinucleated giant cell found in lymphoid tissues, of which the Warthin–Finkeldey giant cell of measles is the paradigm. These cells can be found in lymph nodes in association with a variety of reactive and neoplastic disorders. They measure 25–150 μm in diameter and have as many as 60 nuclei arranged in grape vine clusters. Their cytoplasm is very scanty. Although some early studies suggested a T cell phenotype, more recent evaluations are in keeping with the hypothesis that these cells are multinucleated forms of follicular dendritic cells, a possibility that fits much better their morphologic appearance.

Inflammatory/hyperplastic Diseases

Acute Nonspecific Lymphadenitis

The typical case of acute nonspecific lymphadenitis is rarely biopsied. Microscopically, the earliest change is sinus dilation resulting from increased flow of lymph, followed by accumulation of neutrophils, vascular dilation, and edema of the capsule. *Suppurative lymphadenitis* is a feature of staphylococcal infection, mesenteric lymphadenitis, and cat-scratch disease. *Necrotizing features* may be seen in bubonic plague, tularemia, anthrax, typhoid fever, melioidosis, and the entity known as Kikuchi necrotizing lymphadenitis.

Chronic Nonspecific Lymphadenitis

The morphologic features and the concept of chronic lymphadenitis merge with those of hyperplasia. The general features of chronic lymphadenitis are follicular hyperplasia; prominence of postcapillary venules; increased number of immunoblasts, plasma cells, and histiocytes; and fibrosis. The capsule may appear inflamed and/or fibrotic, and the process may extend into the immediate perinodal tissues. In some cases, one may find an undue predominance in the number of eosinophils, foamy macrophages, and/or mast cells. Terms such as *eosinophilic* or *xanthogranulomatous lymphadenitis* have been sometimes used, depending on the type of the infiltrate. The presence of numerous eosinophils in a lymph node should raise the possibility of Langerhans cell histiocytosis, parasitic infections, Hodgkin lymphoma, autoimmune disorders, and Kimura disease. Eosinophils can also be numerous in epithelioid hemangioma/angiolymphoid hyperplasia with eosinophilia (which may rarely involve lymph nodes), Churg–Strauss disease, and anaplastic large cell lymphoma.

Tuberculosis

Lymph nodes involved by tuberculosis may become adherent to each other and form a large multinodular mass that can be confused clinically with metastatic carcinoma. The most common location of clinically apparent lymphadenopathy is the cervical region ('scrofula'), where a draining sinus that communicates with the skin ('scrofuloderma') may form. Microscopically, the appearance ranges from multiple small epithelioid granulomas reminiscent of sarcoidosis to huge caseous masses surrounded by

Langhans giant cells, epithelioid cells, and lymphocytes. Demonstration of the organisms by special stains, cultures, or PCR is necessary to establish the diagnosis.

Atypical Mycobacteriosis

Atypical mycobacteria are a common cause of granulomatous lymphadenitis. In the United States, caseating granulomatous disease in a cervical lymph node of a child unaccompanied by pulmonary involvement is more likely to be caused by an atypical mycobacterium. The process typically involves lateral nodes in the midportion of the neck. Drainage may continue for months or years in the absence of specific therapy, and healing may result in scarring and contractures. Microscopically, the host reaction may be indistinguishable from that of tuberculosis, but often the granulomatous response is overshadowed by suppurative changes. A nontuberculous mycobacterial etiology should also be suspected if the granulomas are ill-defined (nonpalisading), irregularly shaped, or serpiginous. An acid-fast stain should be performed in every granulomatous and suppurative lymphadenitis of unknown etiology, especially if the patient is a child or an HIV-infected individual. The final identification of the organism rests on the cultural or molecular characteristics.

In immunosuppressed patients, mycobacterial infections may result in a florid spindle cell proliferation that can simulate a neoplastic process (*mycobacterial spindle cell pseudotumor*).

Sarcoidosis

The enigmatic clinicopathologic entity known as sarcoidosis has a worldwide distribution. Scandinavian countries are particularly affected. In the United States, the disease is 10–15 times more common in blacks than in whites. Practically every organ can be involved, but the ones most commonly affected are lung, lymph nodes, eyes, skin, and liver. Erythema nodosum often precedes or accompanies the disease. Functional hypoparathyroidism is the rule, although a few cases of sarcoidosis coexisting with primary hyperparathyroidism have also been reported. This seems to be due to the secretion of a parathyroid hormone (PTH)-related protein by the cells in the granuloma.

Microscopically, the basic lesion is a small granuloma mainly composed of epithelioid cells, with scattered Langhans giant cells and lymphocytes. As a general rule, the Langhans giant cells are smaller and have fewer nuclei than those typically seen in tuberculosis. Necrosis is either absent or limited to a small central fibrinoid focus ('hard' granulomas); a 'necrotizing' variant of sarcoidosis exists, but this is usually extranodal. Schaumann bodies, asteroid bodies, and calcium oxalate crystals are sometimes found in the cytoplasm of the giant cells. Schaumann bodies are round, have concentric laminations, and contain iron and calcium. Ultrastructurally, asteroid bodies are composed of radiating filamentous arms enveloped by 'myelonoid' membranes. Elemental analysis has shown calcium, phosphorus, silicon, and aluminum in these formations. Peculiar PAS-positive inclusions known as Hamazaki-Wesenberg, yellow, or ovoid bodies were claimed to be specific for sarcoidosis, but subsequent histochemical and ultrastructural studies have shown that they have no etiologic or pathogenetic significance. They probably represent large lysosomes containing hemolipofuscin material and are found in a large variety of conditions. None of these inclusions is specific for sarcoidosis. As a matter of fact, from a pathologic standpoint the diagnosis of sarcoidosis is always one of exclusion. A noncaseating granulomatous inflammation in the lymph nodes or skin microscopically indistinguishable from sarcoidosis can be seen in tuberculosis, atypical mycobacteriosis (including swimming pool granuloma), fungus diseases, leprosy, syphilis, leishmaniasis, brucellosis, tularemia, chalazion, zirconium granuloma, berylliosis, Crohn disease, Hodgkin lymphoma; in nodes draining a carcinoma; and in several other conditions. Only when all these possibilities have been excluded and the clinical picture is characteristic is there justification in labeling a case as consistent with sarcoidosis.

Most of the lymphocytes present in the sarcoidal granulomas are T cells with the helper phenotype; both these cells and the epithelioid histiocytes exhibit features of proliferation and/or activation, as shown by their immunocytochemical positivity with the Ki-67 antibody and for interleukin-1, respectively. Pathogenetically, sarcoidosis is thought to represent a dysfunction of circulating T cells with overactivity of B cells. The association of particular human leukocyte antigens (HLAs) with sarcoidosis suggests a role for HLA-linked immune response genes and disease susceptibility.

The Kveim test for sarcoidosis is an intradermal reaction that occurs following inoculation with an extract of human spleen involved with the disease. It is positive in 60–85% of patients with sarcoidosis, and the number of false-positive results is small. The test is regarded as positive when a biopsy of the area taken 4–6 weeks after inoculation shows microscopically sarcoid-type granuloma.

Fungal Infections

Fungal infections of lymph nodes may present as chronic suppurative lesions, as granulomatous processes, or as a combination of the two. The most important fungal lymphadenitis is *histoplasmosis*, which in addition to the previously mentioned patterns can also result in widespread nodal necrosis and in marked diffuse hyperplasia of sinus histiocytes. Other fungal diseases known to result in lymphadenitis are blastomycosis, paracoccidioidomycosis, coccidioidomycosis, and sporotrichosis. To these, one should add opportunistic infections such as cryptococcosis, aspergillosis, mucormycosis, and candidiasis.

The fungal organisms can usually be demonstrated with Gomorimethenamine-silver (GMS) or PAS–Gridley stains, but sometimes their number is so small that they can be detected only in cultures or by molecular testing.

Toxoplasmosis

Toxoplasmosis, one of the most common parasitic infections of humans and other warm-blooded animals, is caused by the protozoan parasite *Toxoplasma gondii*. Toxoplasmic lymphadenitis (formerly known as Piringer–Kuchinka lymphadenitis), in its most typical form, involves the posterior cervical nodes of young women. On palpation, the nodes are firm and only moderately enlarged. Microscopically, the nodal architecture is rather well preserved. The typical triad of the disease, which, however, is not present in all cases, is constituted by: (1) marked follicular hyperplasia, associated with intense mitotic activity and phagocytosis of nuclear debris; (2) small granulomas composed almost entirely of epithelioid cells, located within the hyperplastic follicles and at the periphery, encroaching on and blurring their margins; and (3) distention of marginal and cortical sinuses by monocytoid B cells. An additional feature is the presence of immunoblasts and plasma cells in the medullary cords. Variations on the theme include presence in the granulomas of necrosis or more than an occasional Langhans giant cell.

If the diagnosis of toxoplasmic lymphadenitis is suspected from the microscopic pattern, it should be confirmed serologically, keeping in mind, however, that these tests may be normal in the early stages of the disease.

The differential diagnosis of toxoplasmosis includes other infectious diseases and the lymphocyte predominant form of Hodgkin lymphoma. The collections of epithelioid cells *within* germinal centers seems to be a nearly specific feature for toxoplasmosis.

Syphilis

Generalized lymphadenopathy is a common finding in secondary syphilis, whereas localized node enlargement can be seen in the primary and tertiary stages of the disease. In secondary syphilis, the changes are those of a florid follicular hyperplasia. In primary syphilis, the combination of changes may result in a mistaken diagnosis of malignant lymphoma. Most of the cases have presented as solitary inguinal lymphadenopathy. There are capsular and pericapsular inflammation and extensive fibrosis, diffuse plasma cell infiltration, proliferation of blood vessels with endothelium swelling and inflammatory infiltration of their wall, and follicular hyperplasia. Rarely, noncaseating granulomas and abscesses are present. Exceptionally, the appearance is that of a nodal inflammatory pseudotumor, the message being that spirochetes should be searched for whenever making that diagnosis in a nodal biopsy, by histochemical or immunohistochemical stain.

The morphologic features of syphilitic infection are not substantially different when occurring in HIV-infected patients and can be identified in most cases by the Warthin–Starry or Levaditi stains, by immunofluorescence techniques applied to imprint preparations, or immunohistochemical staining on paraffin section. The organisms are most frequently found in the wall of blood vessels. Detection of *Treponema pallidum* is now also feasible in lymph node biopsies and fine needle aspirations by PCR and Southern blotting.

Leprosy

Lymph nodes involved by the lepromatous type of leprosy have a very characteristic microscopic appearance. The main change is the progressive accumulation of large, pale, rounded histiocytes ('lepra' or 'Virchow' cells), without granuloma formation and with minimal or no necrosis. Wade-Fite and Fite-Faraco stains (which are modified Ziehl-Nielsen reactions) demonstrate packing of the cytoplasm by acid-fast organisms, which can also be demonstrated by a fluorescent method and with the PCR technique.

Mesenteric Lymphadenitis

Mesenteric lymphadenitis is produced by *Yersinia pseudotuber-culosis* or *Yersinia enterocolitica*, two gram-negative polymorphic coccoid or ovoid motile organisms. It is a benign, self-limited disease that can clinically simulate acute appendicitis. Microscopically, there are capsular thickening and edema, increase of immunoblasts and plasma cells in the cortical and paracortical region, dilation of sinuses with accumulation of large lymphocytes within, and germinal center hyperplasia. In the lymphadenitis produced by *Yersinia pseudotuberculosis*, small granulomas and abscesses are commonly present, whereas this is unusual in infection caused by *Yersinia enterocolitica*. These nodal changes are accompanied by inflammatory changes of the terminal ileum and cecum. Ideally, the diagnosis should be confirmed with cultures. Too often, the diagnosis of mesenteric lymphadenitis is made on normal or mildly hyperplastic nodes in an attempt to explain why a patient with the clinical picture of acute appendicitis has a normal appendix.

The organism can be identified with PCR techniques. Interestingly, pathogenetic *Yersinia* DNA has been detected in mesenteric lymph nodes in patients with Crohn disease.

Cat-scratch Disease

Cat-scratch disease is characterized by a primary cutaneous lesion and enlargement of regional lymph nodes, usually axillary or cervical. The changes in the nodes vary with time. Early lesions have histiocytic proliferation and follicular hyperplasia, intermediate lesions have granulomatous changes, and late lesions have abscesses of various sizes. These abscesses are very suggestive of the diagnosis because of their pattern of central, sometimes stellate necrosis with neutrophils, surrounded by a palisading of histiocytes. However, similar abscesses can be seen in lymphogranuloma venereum. Another common feature of lymph nodes with cat-scratch disease is the packing of sinuses by monocytoid B cells, which, together with the follicular hyperplasia, may simulate toxoplasmosis. However, clusters of perifollicular and intrafollicular epithelioid cells are absent.

The primary lesion is a red papule in the skin at the site of inoculation, usually appearing between 7 and 12 days following contact. It may become pustular or crusted. Microscopically, there are foci of necrosis in the dermis surrounded by a mantle of histiocytes. Multinucleated giant cells, lymphocytes, and eosinophils are also present.

The agent of cat-scratch disease is a coccobacillary pleomorphic extracellular bacterium that can be identified with the Warthin–Starry silver stain, particularly in those cases exhibiting extensive necrosis. This organism, which has also been detected ultrastructurally, was originally designated *Rochalimaea henselae* and has been renamed *Bartonella henselae*. The diagnosis can be confirmed by serology, immunohistochemistry, or PCR.

Rare complications of the disease include granulomatous conjunctivitis, thrombocytopenic purpura, and central nervous system manifestations.

Lymphogranuloma venereum

This sexually transmitted disease (not to be confused with granuloma inguinale) is caused by *Chlamydia trachomatis* organisms corresponding to serotypes L1, L2, and L3. The initial lesion is a small (2–3 mm), painless genital vesicle or ulcer which often goes unnoticed and heals in a few days. This is followed by inguinal adenopathy, which can be very prominent. The earliest microscopic change in an affected node is represented by tiny necrotic foci infiltrated by neutrophils. These enlarge and coalesce to form the stellate abscess that represents the most characteristic feature of this disease. In later stages, epithelioid cells, scattered Langhans giant cells, and fibroblasts are seen to line the abscesses' walls. Confluence of these abscesses is common, and cutaneous sinus tracts may develop. The healing stage is represented by nodules with dense fibrous walls surrounding amorphous material.

The microscopic picture just described is not pathognomonic of this disease. Similar changes can occur in cat-scratch disease, atypical mycobacteriosis, and tularemia. Therefore a presumptive diagnosis of lymphogranuloma venereum should be confirmed with the Frei test, complement fixation, immunofluorescence, or molecular testing.

Tularemia

Tularemia is a bacterial disease produced by *Francisella tularensis*, an extremely virulent pathogen, which has recently gained notoriety as a potential biowarfare agent. In the ulcero-glandular form of the disease, prominent lymphadenopathy occurs; this predominates in the axillary region when mammalian vectors are involved and in cervical or inguinal regions with arthropod vectors. A history of handling rabbits suggests the diagnosis in the first instance. The diagnosis is supported by a rise in hemagglutinin titers. Microscopically, the picture in the acute phase is that of an intense lymphadenitis with widespread necrosis, sometimes associated with irregularly shaped microabscesses and granulomas. In the more chronic forms, there is a granulomatous reaction that in some cases may have a frankly tuberculosis-like appearance.

Brucellosis

Brucellosis is caused by *Brucella abortus, melitensis,* or *suis.* In the United States it has evolved from an occupational to a foodborne illness related to consumption of milk and cheese. The most common clinical manifestations are fever, hepatomegaly, and splenomegaly. Lymphadenopathy is uncommon and, when present, usually of modest dimensions. Microscopically, there may be nonspecific follicular hyperplasia and clusters of epithelioid histiocytes sometimes forming large noncaseating granulomas. This is accompanied by a polymorphic infiltrate containing eosinophils, plasma cells, and immunoblasts. When the latter are numerous, the microscopic picture may show a vague resemblance to Hodgkin lymphoma.

AIDS-related Lymphadenopathy

The lymph node abnormalities in AIDS patients can be of various types. They include mycobacterial and other opportunistic infections (some resulting in spindle cell pseudotumors), Kaposi sarcoma, malignant lymphomas of either Hodgkin or non-Hodgkin type, and *florid reactive hyperplasia.* The latter change is the most common. It may be accompanied by collections of monocytoid B cells in the sinuses, neutrophils, and features of dermatopathic lymphadenopathy. In many of the cases, the reactive germinal centers show a feature termed *follicle lysis,* characterized by invagination of mantle lymphocytes into the germinal centers. This is associated with disruption of these centers ('moth-eaten appearance') and a distinctive clustering of large follicular center cells, resulting in an appearance that has been termed *explosive follicular hyperplasia.* Ultrastructurally, a prominence of follicular dendritic cells exhibiting alterations of their fine processes has been described; it has been suggested also on the basis of immunohistochemically (fascin stain) that the AIDS virus preferentially infects these cells. It has been suggested that the polykaryocytes (Warthin-Finkeldey cells) that are sometimes seen in HIV-infected nodes are a multinucleated form of follicular dendritic cell. Immunohistochemically, positive stain for the HIV core protein P24 has been documented within the abnormal germinal centers.

Some lymph nodes in AIDS patients may also show advanced lymphocyte depletion, with or without abnormal (regressively transformed) germinal centers.

The interfollicular tissue may show prominent vascular proliferation, the resulting picture acquiring a vague resemblance to Castleman disease. It is important to search in these areas and in the subcapsular region for the earliest signs of development of Kaposi sarcoma. These changes should be distinguished from those of vascular transformation of the sinuses.

A rough relationship has been found among the pattern of nodal reaction, the cell suspension immunophenotypic data, and the patient's HIV status.

The term *chronic lymphadenopathy syndrome* has been defined as an unexplained enlargement of nodes of at least 3 months' duration at two or more extrainguinal sites in an individual at risk for AIDS. The microscopic picture is similar to that described previously. Overall, up to a fourth of the patients have developed AIDS on follow-up, cachexia and weight loss being the clinical signs of this progression.

Infectious Mononucleosis

The etiologic agent of classic infectious mononucleosis is the EBV, but other agents may be involved in atypical cases. It is rare for the pathologist to see a lymph node from a patient with a typical clinical picture because in most instances the presumptive clinical diagnosis is confirmed by examination of the peripheral blood and serologic evaluation without need of a lymph node biopsy. It is in the atypical case, presenting with lymphadenopathy without fever, sore throat, or splenomegaly, that the clinician will perform a lymph node biopsy to rule out the possibility of malignant lymphoma.

Microscopically, nodes and other lymphoid organs affected by infectious mononucleosis can be confused with malignant lymphoma because of the effacement of the architecture; infiltration of the trabecula, capsule, and perinodal fat; and the marked proliferation of immunoblasts, immature plasma cells, and mature plasma cells ('polymorphic B cell hyperplasia'). These features are particularly prominent when the disease develops in transplant recipients or other immunosuppressed patients. Necrosis may also be present; this is usually only focal but in immunodeficient children it may be massive.

Features of importance in the differential diagnosis with lymphoma include the predominantly sinusal distribution of the large lymphoid cells, follicular hyperplasia with marked mitotic activity and phagocytosis (these follicles being usually small), increase in the number of plasma cells, and vascular proliferation. Another important feature is the fact that, although the nodal architecture may appear effaced, the sinusal pattern remains intact or even focally accentuated, a fact appreciated particularly well with reticulin stains. Another supposedly characteristic feature of this disease is the presence in the sinuses of clusters or 'colonies' of lymphocytes in graduated sizes, from the small lymphocyte to the large lymphoid cell or immunoblast. The latter cell usually has only one large vesicular nucleus with a thin nuclear membrane and one or two prominent amphophilic or basophilic nucleoli. A paranuclear 'hof' is often seen. When binucleated, this cell may closely resemble a Reed-Sternberg cell and result in a mistaken diagnosis of Hodgkin lymphoma. Immunophenotyping evaluation should resolve the issue in most cases, despite the existence of an overlap that may be providing a pathogenetic insight into the nature and possible relationship of these two disorders. The diagnosis of infectious mononucleosis can be confirmed by *in situ* hybridization techniques.

Langerhans Cell Histiocytosis

The terms Langerhans cell histiocytosis (LCH), Langerhans cell granulomatosis, histiocytosis X, differentiated histiocytosis, and eosinophilic granuloma are applied to a specific, although remarkably variable, clinicopathologic entity characterized and defined by the proliferation of Langerhans cells. These cells are regarded as a distinct type of immune 'accessory' cells that are involved in the capturing of some antigens and their presentation to the lymphoid cells. Contrary to a formerly held belief, these cells are not primarily phagocytic in nature. Their nuclei are highly characteristic: Irregular, usually elongated, with prominent grooves and folds that traverse them in all directions. The cytoplasm is abundant and acidophilic, sometimes to the point that an embryonal rhabdomyosarcoma is simulated. Most Langerhans cells are mononuclear, but occasional ones contain several nuclei while still maintaining the aforementioned nuclear and cytoplasmic features. Histochemically, they show weak acid phosphatase and nonspecific esterase activity but considerable leucyl-β-naphthylamidase activity and membrane-bound ATPase activity. They are believed to develop from a lymphoid-committed precursor, a hypothesis supported by the presence of an identical rearrangement of the immunoglobulin heavy chain gene in a case we studied which had both neoplastic Langerhans cells and B lymphocytes (Box 1).

Box 1: Pathologic staging of Langerhans cell histiocytosis (histiocyte society)

A   Bone only or bone with involvement of first echelon lymph nodes in drainage field (osteolymphatic disease) and/or contiguous soft tissue involvement

    A1 Monostotic

    A2 Monostotic with osteolymphatic disease

    A3 Monostotic with contiguous soft tissue involvement

    A4 Polyostotic

    A5 Polyostotic with osteolymphatic disease

    A6 Polyostotic with contiguous soft tissue involvement

B   Skin and/or other squamous mucous membranes only or with involvement of related superficial lymph nodes

    B1 Nodular disease; neonatal period without nodal disease

    B2 Nodular disease; neonatal period with nodal disease

    B3 Multiple nodules or diffuse maculopapular disease without nodal disease

    B4 Multiple nodules or diffuse maculopapular disease with nodal disease

C   Soft tissue and viscera only excluding above and multisystem disease. Specify tissue involved, e.g. lung, lymph node, brain

D   Multisystem disease with any combination of the above. Specify each organ/tissue involved, e.g. skin, bone marrow, bone

From Warnke RA, Weiss LM, Chan JKC, Cleary ML, Dorfman RF. Tumors of the lymph nodes and spleen. Atlas of tumor pathology, series 3, fascicle 14. Washington, DC, 1995, Armed Forces Institute of Pathology.

Lymph node involvement can be seen as a component of the systemic form, or it may represent the initial and sometimes exclusive manifestation of the disease. The microscopic appearance is characteristic. There is distention of the sinuses by an infiltrate of mononuclear and multinuclear Langerhans cells, admixed with a variable number of eosinophils; foci of necrosis are common, often surrounded by a rim of eosinophils (so-called 'eosinophilic microabscesses'), and always confined to the sinuses. The nodal architecture may be preserved or variably effaced.

Sometimes, incidental foci of LCH are seen in lymph nodes involved by non-Hodgkin lymphoma or Hodgkin lymphoma, a sharp segregation existing between the two processes. In most of these cases, the Langerhans cell proliferation is limited to the node and may represent a reaction to the lymphoma, but in others it is an expression of generalized LCH. Follow-up studies have shown a broad spectrum of involvement, embracing all those syndromes that have been associated with LCH. However, the prognosis is usually excellent.

Malignant Lymphoma

Malignant lymphoma is the generic term given to tumors of the lymphoid system and specifically of lymphocytes and their precursor cells, whether of T, B, or null phenotypes. Although traditionally tumors presumed to be composed of histiocytes and other cells of the accessory immune system have also been included in the category of malignant lymphoma, it would seem more appropriate to regard them separately for both conceptual and practical reasons. Such tumors undoubtedly exist, and are discussed later in this chapter. One should be aware, however, that the large majority of tumors that were designated in the past as histiocytic lymphomas or reticulum cell sarcomas are in reality of lymphocytic nature and therefore true malignant lymphomas.

Although some overlapping exists, the term *malignant lymphoma* is reserved for those neoplastic processes that initially present as localized lesions and are characterized by the formation of gross tumor nodules. Conversely, neoplastic lymphoid proliferations that are systemic and diffuse from their inception are included among the leukemias.

The malignant lymphomas can be divided into two major categories: Hodgkin lymphoma and all the others, which, for lack of a better term, are known collectively as non-Hodgkin lymphomas. Both groups are further subdivided into several more or less distinct subcategories, the classification currently in vogue being that proposed by the World Health Organization. This classification has incorporated a wealth of information gathered from the fields of immunohistochemistry, molecular genetics, genomics, and proteomics. The results have been spectacular, but unfortunately they have resulted in calling into question the role of traditional histologic examination in lymphoma diagnosis. As several of the most accomplished hematopathologists have pointed out in sharp editorials and essays, that role is, and is likely to remain, critical.

Hodgkin Lymphoma

The disease originally described by Thomas Hodgkin in 1832 and which Samuel Wilks first proposed to be called Hodgkin disease makes one of the richest chapters of history of oncologic pathology.

The conventional definition of Hodgkin disease—a very ingrained term that the World Health Organization (WHO) Committee has replaced by that of Hodgkin lymphoma—is that of a type of malignant lymphoma in which Reed-Sternberg cells are present in a 'characteristic background' of reactive inflammatory cells of various types, accompanied by fibrosis of a variable degree. Thus identification of typical Reed-Sternberg cells is necessary for the initial diagnosis of Hodgkin lymphoma (except for NLPHL, *see* below). As far as the 'characteristic background' or 'appropriate milieu' is concerned, it is highly variable, but it lacks the monomorphic appearance of most other malignant lymphomas (again with the exception of NLPHL). Mature lymphocytes, eosinophils, plasma cells, and histiocytes may all be present in greater or lesser amount, depending on the microscopic type. Many of the Reed-Sternberg cells are surrounded by T lymphocytes arranged in a rosette-like fashion.

The etiology of Hodgkin lymphoma remains unknown, but there is considerable evidence to suggest that the EBV plays an important role. Individuals with a history of infectious mononucleosis have an increased incidence of Hodgkin lymphoma; patients with Hodgkin lymphoma have an altered antibody pattern to EBV prior to diagnosis; marked phenotypic similarities exist between infectious mononucleosis and Hodgkin lymphoma; and EBV genomes have been identified in Reed-Sternberg cells in up to half of the cases (particularly in the mixed cellularity subtype, in young patients, and/or in developing countries). There is also evidence for a genetic susceptibility factor.

Gross Features

Except for the very early stages, lymph nodes involved by Hodgkin lymphoma are enlarged, sometimes massively so. The gross appearance is somewhat dependent on the microscopic subtypes. The consistency varies from soft to hard depending on the amount of fibrosis. Some degree of nodularity is often appreciated, particularly in the nodular sclerosis form. Foci of necrosis may be present. Except for NLPHL, the cut surface of the node has a more heterogeneous appearance than most non-Hodgkin lymphomas. In advanced cases, several nodes from the same group become matted together, a feature spectacularly demonstrated in the drawing that accompanied Hodgkin's classic article.

Reed-Sternberg Cell

The classic Reed-Sternberg cell, as seen in all subtypes of classic Hodgkin lymphoma (but not in NLPHL, *see* below), is a large cell (20–50 μm in diameter or more) with abundant weakly acidophilic or amphophilic cytoplasm, which may appear homogeneous or granular and which lacks a pale zone in the Golgi area. The nucleus is bilobed or polylobed so that the cell appears binucleated or multinucleated; it is possible that in some cases bona fide binucleation or multinucleation actually occurs. The nuclear membrane is thick and sharply defined. The nuclear pattern is usually vesicular but with some coarse chromatin clumps scattered throughout. There is a very large, variously shaped, but usually rounded, highly acidophilic central nucleolus surrounded by a clear halo. In the most typical example of the Reed-Sternberg cell, the two nuclear lobes face each other ('mirror image'), resulting in the oft-cited 'owl eye' appearance. When multilobation occurs, the appearance has been likened to that of an 'egg basket'. Cells with this set of features but lacking nuclear lobation have been referred to as mononuclear variants of Reed-Sternberg cells or Hodgkin cells. Although their presence should suggest the possibility of Hodgkin lymphoma, they are not diagnostic by themselves. It has been stated that the minimal requirement for a diagnostic Reed-Sternberg cell is a bilobed nucleus in which at least one of the lobes has a prominent acidophilic nucleolus. At the other end of this spectrum is the Reed-Sternberg cell of giant size and highly pleomorphic hyperchromatic nuclei, having an appearance such as to simulate the cells of anaplastic carcinoma or one of the pleomorphic sarcomas. Another type of Reed-Sternberg cell, characterized by a darkly staining and retracted quality, is referred to as the mummified or necrobiotic variant and appears to be the morphologic expression of apoptosis. Additional morphologic variations of Reed-Sternberg cells exist, and these will be discussed with the various types of Hodgkin lymphoma.

The Reed-Sternberg cell of Hodgkin lymphoma needs to be distinguished from other multinucleated cells that may be present in lymph nodes. Megakaryocytes can simulate it closely in hematoxylin–eosin stained sections, but they can be identified by the presence of a strongly PAS-positive substance in their cytoplasm and their different immunophenotype, which includes positivity for factor VIII-related antigen and CD61. Cells morphologically very similar to Reed-Sternberg cells, representing pleomorphic immunoblasts, can be seen in infectious mono-nucleosis and other viral diseases. The most important mor-phologic differences between these two cells are summarized in Table 7.6. Neoplastic cells from a variety of epithelial and mesen-chymal tumors also can resemble Reed-Sternberg cells. Finally, some malignant lymphomas of non-Hodgkin type may be accompanied by cells with the appearance of Reed-Sternberg cells, a fact that raises some questions about the very definition of Hodgkin lymphoma and its existence as an entity. In all of these disorders—and especially in the lymphomas—it is of the utmost importance to examine not only the putative Reed-Sternberg cells but also the background in which they are situated. The more cytologically atypical the lymphoid population, the less likely the diagnosis of Hodgkin lymphoma.

The requirement for the presence of classic Reed-Sternberg cells, which is absolute for the initial diagnosis of Hodgkin lymphoma, can be lessened somewhat in subsequent biopsies from patients with documented Hodgkin lymphoma or when the typical immunophenotype can be demonstrated. Under these circums-tances, the presence of a polymorphic infiltrate *with atypical mononuclear cells* but not classic Reed-Sternberg cells in a biopsy of bone marrow, liver, or some other organ can be taken as evidence of involvement by Hodgkin lymphoma; however, a note of caution should be interjected. Atypical large lymphoid cells *need* to be present; an infiltrate of eosinophils, lymphocytes, and plasma cells or a collection of epithelioid granulomas is not enough.

Table 7.6: Major morphologic differences between the pleomorphic immuno-blast (Reed-Sternberg-like cell) of infectious mononucleosis and the Reed-Sternberg cell of Hodgkin lymphoma

Feature	*Immunoblast*	*Reed-Sternberg cell*
Nucleolus		
Staining pattern	Basophilic	Acidophilic
Contours	Irregular	Regular, with clear halo (inclusion-like)
Position	Adjacent to nuclear membrane	More centrally located
Cytoplasm		
Staining pattern	Usually amphophilic	Usually acidophilic
Pyroninophilia	Invariably strong	Variable
Paranuclear hof	Prominent	Inconspicuous
Surrounding cells	Mononuclear immuno-blasts and plasmacytoid cells	Lymphocytes and histiocytes

Compiled from data in Dorfman RF, Warnke R. Lymphadenopathy simulating the malignant lymphomas. Hum Pathol 1974, 5: 519–550.

The nature of the Reed-Sternberg cell has been one of the most controversial issues in pathology. Practically all the cells present in the normal node (and even some that are not) have been proposed at one time or another as possible progenitors, including B cells, T cells, histiocytes, follicular dendritic cells, and inter-digitating dendritic cells, but current evidence indicates that most if not all cases of Hodgkin lymphoma represent neoplasms of B cells (functional B cells for NLPHL, and 'crippled' B cells for classic Hodgkin lymphoma).

The immunocytochemical profile of the Reed-Sternberg cell in classic Hodgkin lymphoma is yet to be totally agreed upon because of the discrepancies among the various laboratories, which may be due to technical factors or to the heterogeneity of the disease, which sometimes manifests itself in sequential biopsies of the same case. The most important results in paraffin-embedded material are the following:

• CD15 (Leu-M1): This is expressed in over 80% of the cases; the pattern may be paranuclear (corresponding to the Golgi region), diffuse cytoplasmic, and/or related to the cell membrane.

- CD30 (Ki-1): As recognized by the monoclonal antibody Ber-H2, this is found in over 90% of the cases.
- CD45 (LCA): This is expressed in less than 10% of the cases.
- CD45RO and CD43 (T-lineage-related antigens): These are expressed in less than 10% of the cases.
- CD20 (L26, B-lineage antigen): This is expressed in 10–20% of the cases, usually in a heterogeneous pattern, i.e. only a fraction of Reed-Sternberg cells are positive and stain with variable intensities.
- PAX5, a B cell transcription factor, is positive in most cases, supporting the B-lineage of Reed-Sternberg cells. However, the intensity of staining is often weak to moderate compared with normal B cells. This marker is of great help for distinguishing classic Hodgkin lymphoma from anaplastic large cell lymphoma (PAX5 negative).
- CD40 (a protein present in B cells and nerve growth factor receptor): This is expressed in approximately 70%.
- CD74: This is expressed in over 75%.
- Fascin: This is an actin-bundling protein which is normally expressed by dendritic cells. This unexpected observation, coupled with the report of a subset of cases of Hodgkin lymphoma in which the Reed–Sternberg cells stained for CD21 (another dendritic follicular cell marker) but not for any B cell marker, is intriguing and not exactly in line with the prevailing hypothesis about the nature of these cells.
- Restin (an intermediate filament-associated protein): This is present in approximately 80%. The same is true for anaplastic large cell lymphoma but not for other types of non-Hodgkin lymphoma.
- Peanut agglutinin and *Bauhinia purpurea* lectins: They are expressed in over 60% of the cases, in contrast to their near universal absence in non-Hodgkin lymphoma.
- Others, such as CD95 (a member of the superfamily that includes the nerve growth factor and tumor necrosis factors receptors, TNFRs) and its ligand, the factor associated to TNFRs, Fas ligand, granzyme B (a serine protease expressed by activated cytotoxic T cells and NK cells), and TARC (a lymphocyte-directed CC chemokine that attracts activated T-helper type 2 cells).

In frozen sections, a large percentage of Reed-Sternberg cells have been found to exhibit reactivity for one or more pan-T cell or pan-B cell antigens, including the framework antigen of the T cell receptor β chain. They also express polyclonal IgG (probably representing passive uptake via the Fc receptor), HLA-DR, CD25 (the interleukin-2 receptor), and CD71 (the transferrin receptor).

Molecular studies have also given rise to controversial results. Most cases of Hodgkin lymphoma yield a germline configuration for immunoglobulin heavy and light chain genes and the β T cell receptor genes, but this simply results from a dilution factor by the non-neoplastic cells; indeed, some studies suggest that an increased number of Reed-Sternberg cells and their variants is associated with a detectable increase in clonal rearrangements of either gene. In a remarkable experiment, Reed-Sternberg cells were isolated from 12 cases of 'classic' Hodgkin lymphoma and found to have rearranged immunoglobulin variable-region heavy-chain (V_H) genes, indicating their origin from B cells. In half of the cases the population of Reed–Sternberg cells was polyclonal, and in the other half it was monoclonal or mixed. Several other workers have provided additional evidence in favor of the interpretation that Reed-Sternberg cells derive from mature B cells at the germinal center stage of differentiation, although some discordant hard-to-explain findings persist. In contrast with anaplastic large cell lymphoma, there is no t(2;5) translocation.

Another controversial issue is the prevalence of t(14;18) in Hodgkin lymphoma, the reported figures ranging from zero to over 30%; perhaps of significance in this regard is the fact that the BCL2 protein (a hallmark of the 14;18 translocation) is never overexpressed, except in those exceptional instances of Hodgkin lymphoma that arise in the setting of follicular lymphoma.

Overexpression of the P53 product as detected immuno-histochemically is common in Hodgkin lymphoma, but it does not correlate with gene mutations, which are rare.

Microscopic Types

For many years, Jackson and Parker's classification of Hodgkin lymphoma into granuloma, paragranuloma, and sarcoma variants was widely used because of its reproducibility and clearcut prognostic implications, the major objection being that too many of the cases (approximately 80%) fell into one of the categories—i.e. Hodgkin granuloma. The concept of a sclerosing type of Hodgkin lymphoma associated with a very good prognosis was first introduced by Smetana and Cohen in 1956 and incorporated into a new classification proposed by Lukes et al. In this scheme, six categories were included: Lymphocytic and/or histiocytic (L&H) nodular, L&H diffuse, nodular sclerosis, mixed cellularity, diffuse fibrosis, and reticular. This classification, somewhat simplified and with some changes in nomenclature (not always for the better), was adopted by the Nomenclature Committee at the Rye Conference on Hodgkin lymphoma. This classification recognized four major types of Hodgkin lymphoma: nodular sclerosis, lymphocyte predominance, lymphocyte depletion, and mixed cellularity. In the REAL/WHO scheme currently in use there has been a further reshuffling of the types into two major categories: The nodular subtype of lymphocyte predominant and the classic, the latter incorporating all other types of the Rye classification. The relationships between these classifications are shown in Table 7.7.

Table 7.7: Comparison between the different classifications of Hodgkin lymphoma proposed over the years

Jackson and Parker (1947)	Smetana and Cohen's Addition (1956)	Lukes (1963)	Rye Conference (1966)	REAL/WHO (2001/2008)
Paragranuloma	Paragranuloma	Lymphocytic and histiocytic, nodular	Lymphocyte predominant	Nodular lymphocyte predominant
		Lymphocytic and histiocytic, diffuse		Classic, lymphocyte-rich subtype
Granuloma	Granuloma	Mixed cellularity	Mixed cellularity	Classic, mixed cellularity subtype
	Nodular sclerosis	Nodular sclerosis	Nodular sclerosis	Classic, nodular sclerosis subtype
Sarcoma	Sarcoma	Diffuse fibrosis and reticular	Lymphocyte depletion	Classic, lymphocyte depletion subtype

Nodular Lymphocyte Predominant Hodgkin Lymphoma

In **nodular lymphocyte predominant** Hodgkin lymphoma (NLPHL), the predominant cell is a small B lymphocyte, with or without an accompanying population of benign-appearing histiocytes. Postcapillary venules with high endothelium may be prominent. The lymph node architecture is partially or totally effaced, and the infiltrate has a variously well-developed nodular pattern of growth. The nodularity may be so pronounced as to simulate on low power the appearance of follicular lymphoma; however, the nodules of NLPHL are more irregular in size and staining quality, and the admixture of lymphocytes and epithelioid cells gives them a mottled appearance. A rim of uninvolved or hyperplastic lymphoid tissue may be present. Progressively transformed germinal centers may be seen adjacent to the lesion. Eosinophils, plasma cells, and foci of fibrosis are scanty or absent. Classic Reed-Sternberg cells are absent. One sees instead a variable but usually large number of a type of Reed-Sternberg cell (the L&H cell, LP cell, or 'popcorn' cell) characterized by a folded, multilobed nucleus with smaller nucleoli. These cells are most commonly found within the nodules. If numerous typical Reed-Sternberg cells are found in a node with a lymphocyte pre-dominant background, the case probably belongs in the classic category (lymphocyte-rich subtype). Occasionally, the L&H cells predominate at the margins of the nodules, creating a 'wreath' around them. In others, they may cluster in large confluent sheets resembling diffuse large cell lymphoma.

Classic Hodgkin Lymphoma

This category, which subsumes all types of Hodgkin lymphoma except for NLPHL, is regarded as a nosologic entity because of the similar immunophenotype of the tumor cells. The differences consist in sites of involvement, clinical features, growth pattern, presence of fibrosis, composition of cellular background, number and degree of atypia of the tumor cells, and prevalence of EBV infection. These subtypes are nodular sclerosis, mixed cellularity, lymphocyte rich, and lymphocyte depletion.

Nodular sclerosis: Hodgkin lymphoma is characterized in its fully developed stage by broad collagen bands separating the lymphoid tissue in well-defined nodules. These fibrous bands, which have a birefringent quality when examined under polarized light, often center around blood vessels. In addition to the classic Reed-Sternberg cell, nodular sclerosis Hodgkin lymphoma also displays a variant known as *lacunar* or *cytoplasmic*. This cell type is quite large (40–50 μm in diameter), with an abundant clear cytoplasm and multilobulated nuclei having complicated in foldings and nucleoli of smaller size than those of the classic Reed-Sternberg cell. The 'frail' cytoplasm of these cells is retracted close to the nuclear membrane so that the cell appears to be floating in a 'lacuna'. This is the result of an artifact induced by formalin fixation, in as much as it is absent in tissues fixed in B5 or Zenker. In some cases, there is clustering of these lacunar cells, particularly around areas of necrosis. They form sheets and cohesive nests, to the point that a mistaken diagnosis of large cell non-Hodgkin lymphoma, carcinoma, germ cell tumor, or thymoma can be made. Cases of nodular sclerosis Hodgkin lymphoma showing prominence of this feature have been referred to as the *syncytial, sarcomatoid,* or *sarcomatous* variant.

Some workers regard the lacunar variant of Reed-Sternberg cells as more typical of this type of Hodgkin lymphoma than the fibrosis itself and make the diagnosis of nodular sclerosis Hodgkin lymphoma in the presence of lacunar cells even if fibrosis is totally lacking (so-called *cellular phase*), however, it should be remarked that lacunar cells are not pathognomonic of this condition. They can also be seen in mixed cellularity Hodgkin lymphoma and even in reactive disorders.

The composition of the non-neoplastic infiltrate varies widely, to the point that some authors have proposed to subdivide nodular sclerosis Hodgkin lymphoma into lymphocyte predominant, mixed cellularity, and lymphocyte depletion categories, and have claimed that this subdivision carries some prognostic implications. Along similar lines, the British National Lymphoma Investigation group has proposed to divide cases of nodular sclerosis Hodgkin lymphoma into two grades. In their scheme, cases are assigned to the allegedly more aggressive grade II if any of these features are present: (1) a 'reticular' or 'pleomorphic' pattern of lymphocytic depletion in over 25% of the cellular nodules; (2) a 'fibrohistiocytic' pattern of lymphocyte depletion in over 80% of the cellular nodules; and (3) the presence of numerous bizarre and highly anaplastic Reed-Sternberg and Hodgkin cells without lymphocyte depletion in over 25% of the nodules. Grade II lesions include the already mentioned 'syncytial' variant of other authors.

In **mixed cellularity** Hodgkin lymphoma, a large number of eosinophils, plasma cells, and atypical mononuclear cells are admixed with classic Reed-Sternberg cells, which tend to be numerous. Focal necrosis may be present, but fibrosis should be minimal or absent. It is somewhat ironic that mixed cellularity Hodgkin lymphoma, which fits more closely the histopathologic picture of the disease as depicted in the classic textbooks, has now almost become a diagnosis of exclusion.

The **lymphocyte-rich** type is characterized by the presence of Reed-Sternberg cells scattered against a nodular (most commonly) or diffuse background, largely composed of small lymphocytes and practically devoid of eosinophils and neutrophils. The main differential diagnosis is with NLPHD, and is primarily based on the presence of cells with the typical morphologic and immuno-histochemical features of Reed-Sternberg cells.

The **lymphocyte-depletion** group, which comprises less than 5% of all cases of Hodgkin lymphoma, includes two morpho-logically different subtypes, designated as 'diffuse fibrosis' and 'reticular' in the original Lukes classification. In the diffuse fibrosis subtype, the number of lymphocytes and other cells progressively decreases as the result of heavy deposition of collagen fibers. The reticular subtype is characterized by a very large number of diagnostic Reed-Sternberg cells (many of them of bizarre con-figuration) among atypical mononuclear cells and other elements. Areas of necrosis are more common than in other types. The 'reticular' subtype of lymphocyte depletion Hodgkin lymphoma needs to be distinguished from non-Hodgkin lymphoma of large cell type (including the anaplastic CD30+ type) and from the variant of nodular sclerosis Hodgkin lymphoma with aggregates of lacunar cells.

Other Microscopic Features

There are some microscopic variations on the theme of Hodgkin lymphoma worth mentioning, mainly because lack of knowledge of their occurrence may result in mistaken diagnoses. These mainly apply to classic Hodgkin lymphoma and its subtypes rather than NLPHL.

1. *Foamy macrophages*: Clumps of foamy macrophages resulting in a xanthogranulomatous appearance may be found, particularly in the nodular sclerosis form.
2. *Eosinophils*: In some instances, the intensity of eosinophilic infiltration is massive and accompanied by so-called 'eosinophilic microabscesses'. Such cases may be confused with Langerhans cell histiocytosis, hypersensitivity reaction, or 'allergic granulomatosis'.
3. *Other inflammatory cells*: S-100 protein-positive dendritic cells, mast cells, and monocytoid B cells may be very numerous.
4. *Focal interfollicular involvement*: In the early stages of the disease, only focal involvement of a lymph node may be encountered,

Table 7.8: Summary of various types of lymphoma with a diffuse mixed cell population

Type	Lineage	Clinical features	Histologic features	Immunohistochemical features	Behavior
Diffuse follicular lymphoma (diffuse centro-blastic–centrocytic)	B	Adults, usually presenting with lymphadenopathy; may have known history of follicular lymphoma or arising *de novo*; disease often at high stage at presentation; extranodal involvement is common	Small cells with angulated (cleaved) or elongated nuclei, fairly condensed chromatin, and scanty cytoplasm; large cells with round or folded nuclei, vesicular chromatin, and multiple distinct nucleoli; neoplastic follicles should be absent; sclerosis common	Pan-B+; CD5–; CD10±; BCL+; may have irregular loose meshworks of follicular dendritic cells	No reliable data in literature on its behavior; some studies suggest that it is low-grade neoplasm, but prognosis is less favorable than for follicular lymphoma
Peripheral T cell lymphoma	T	Usually adults; nodal or extranodal presentation; disease often at high stage at presentation	Prominent high endothelial venules; continuous spectrum of small, medium-sized, and large lymphoid cells; nuclear irregularities, chromatin pattern often granular; clear	Pan-T+ (often with loss of one or more pan-T antigens; usually CD4+, sometimes CD8+, CD4+/ CD8+, or CD4–/CD8–)	Generally aggressive neoplasm

Contd.

Table 7.8: Summary of various types of lymphoma with a diffuse mixed cell population (*Contd.*)

Type	Lineage	Clinical features	Histologic features	Immunohistochemical features	Behavior
			cytoplasm commonly seen in some cells; may show rich component of inflammatory cells (such as eosinophils, histiocytes, and epithelioid cells)		
Lymphoplasma-cytic lymphoma with increased blasts (polymorphic subtype)	B	Usually older adults; nodal or extranodal presentation; may have monoclonal gammopathy (20–40%); disease often disseminated at presentation; occasional cases may have circulating lymphoma cells	Small lymphocytes; lymphoplasmacytoid cells; plasma cells; immunoblasts; rare follicular center cells; Dutcher bodies (nuclear pseudo inclusions of immunoglobulin) may be found; specific lymphoma types should be excluded (e.g. follicular lymphoma, low-grade B cell lymphoma of MALT)	Pan-B+; CD5–; CD10–; CD23–; sIg+, cIg+ (usually IgM type)	Low-grade neoplasm, but prognosis is worse than that of B-SLL/CLL; median survival 55 months; may rarely transform to diffuse large cell lymphoma

Contd.

Table 7.8: Summary of various types of lymphoma with a diffuse mixed cell population (*Contd.*)

Type	Lineage	Clinical features	Histologic features	Immunohistochemical features	Behavior
T cell/histiocyte-rich large B cell lymphoma	B	Older adults, usually presenting with lymphadenopathy; disease often disseminated at presentation	Small lymphocytes with round or irregular nuclei; scattered atypical large cells with round to folded nuclei, distinct nucleoli, and amphophilic cytoplasm; may show rich vascularity and component of inflammatory cells	Large atypical cells: pan-B+; small cells: pan-T+	Aggressive neoplasm; prognosis similar to or worse than conventional diffuse large cell lymphoma
Extranodal marginal zone lymphoma of mucosa-associated lymphoid tissue (MALT)	B	Any age; tumor often localized to mucosal site and/or regional lymph nodes at presentation	Small lymphoid cells with round or irregular nuclei and pale to clear cytoplasm; scattered large blast cells with vesicular nuclei and distinct nucleoli; glandular invasion (lymphoepithelial lesions) common; plasma cells common	Pan-B+; CD5–; CD10–; CD23–	Low-grade neoplasm, with median survival of 8 years; may show late relapse locally or in other mucosal sites; may transform to diffuse large cell lymphoma

Modified from Warnke RA, Weiss LM, Chan JKC, Cleary ML, Dorfman RF. Tumors of the lymph nodes and spleen. Atlas of tumor pathology, series 3, fascicle 14. Washington, DC, 1995, Armed Forces Institute of Pathology.

CLL, chronic lymphocytic leukemia; MALT, mucosa-associated lymphoid tissue; SLL, small lymphocytic lymphoma.

often restricted to the paracortical region between florid hyperplastic follicles; this pattern, which has been referred to as *interfollicular Hodgkin lymphoma,* is not regarded as a specific subtype.

5. *Follicular involvement*: Sometimes the nodal involvement by Hodgkin lymphoma is mainly in the germinal centers, the appearance being reminiscent of NLPHL.

6. *Castleman disease-like features*: Cases of Hodgkin lymphoma may be accompanied or preceded by a plasmacytic infiltrate and abnormalities of germinal centers closely resembling those seen in plasma cell type Castleman disease, probably attributable to interleukin-6 secretion by Reed-Sternberg cells.

7. *Fibrosis*: In cases of nodular sclerosis Hodgkin lymphoma but sometimes also in other types, the amount of fibrosis can be such as to simulate the appearance of one of the inflammatory fibroscleroses (such as sclerosing mediastinitis or retro-peritoneal fibrosis).

8. *Spindle cell proliferation*: In rare cases of Hodgkin lymphoma, there is a proliferation of oval to spindle cells of such a degree as to simulate fibrosarcoma, malignant fibrous histiocytoma, or a follicular dendritic cell tumor; such lesions have been referred to as **fibrosarcomatous or fibroblastic Hodgkin lymphoma**. Some of these spindle cells have a degree of nuclear atypia such as to indicate their neoplastic nature and relationship with Reed-Sternberg and Hodgkin cells; indeed, most of these lesions would be included in the grade II category of nodular sclerosis Hodgkin lymphoma proposed by the British National Lymphoma Investigation Group. Others are of a reactive nature and stromal derivation (i.e. made up of fibroblasts and myofibroblasts).

9. *Noncaseating granulomas*: These formations are sometimes present in nodes and other organs involved by Hodgkin lymphoma. Occasionally they are so numerous as to obscure the diagnostic features of the disease. In other instances, these granulomas may be seen within otherwise uninvolved organs of patients with Hodgkin lymphoma. Their significance is unknown. Perhaps they represent an expression of delayed hypersensitivity. Some seen in the past were reactions to the contrast material used in lymphangiography. Their presence does not indicate involvement of that organ by Hodgkin lymphoma and should therefore not influence the staging

criteria. Actually, it has been suggested that, within a given stage, the presence of these granulomas is associated with a better prognosis.

10. *Vascular invasion*: Blood vessel infiltration has been detected microscopically in 6–14% of the cases of Hodgkin lymphoma by the use of elastic tissue stains. This finding is said to be associated with an increased incidence of extranodal organ involvement, but the statement and the very validity of the observation have been questioned.

Classic Hodgkin Lymphoma

In almost all cases of classic Hodgkin lymphoma, clonal immuno-globulin gene rearrangements can be demonstrated in micro-dissected neoplastic (Reed–Sternberg) cells or tissue samples rich in neoplastic cells; only exceptionally the clonal T cell receptor gene rearrangements are present instead. The variable regions of the immunoglobulin genes frequently show hypermutation but not ongoing mutations. Remarkably, immunoglobulin mRNA transcripts are usually absent, which may result from functional defects in immunoglobulin gene regulatory elements or crippling mutations in the immunoglobulin genes.

About 40% of cases of classic Hodgkin lymphoma are associated with EBV, which can be demonstrated by EBV-LMP1 immuno-histochemistry or EBV-encoded early RNA (EBER) *in situ* hybridization. The association with EBV is stronger at the extremes of age, i.e. children/young adults and elderly adults, and in the mixed cellularity subtype. Of note, the overall frequency of EBV association is much higher in individuals with immunodeficiency (approximately 100%) or from developing countries (80–100%).

Clinical Features

Hodgkin lymphoma comprises approximately 20–30% of all malignant lymphomas in the United States and Western Europe but a much lower percentage in Japan and other Oriental countries. There is a wide range in age incidence, which varies according to geographic location. In the United States, there is a bimodal distribution, with a peak at 15–40 years and a second, smaller peak in the seventh decade. In Japan, the peak in young adulthood is absent. In poorly developed countries, there is a high incidence in children, a relatively low incidence in the 15 to 40-year age group, and a third peak later in life. There is a male preponderance (approximately 1.5:1) in all microscopic types except nodular sclerosis. The disease may present in a variety of ways, the most common (approximately 90% of the cases) being painless enlargement of superficial (usually cervical) lymph nodes. Fever, night sweats, and loss of weight (so-called 'B symptoms') occur in approximately 25% of the cases; their presence influences the clinical staging. Pruritus is also frequent.

Important clinical differences exist related to the microscopic types. The typical patient with NLPHL is a man in his forties with involvement of the high cervical nodes. This microscopic form uncommonly involves the spleen, liver, or bone marrow except when it changes to a more aggressive histologic pattern.

Nodular sclerosis is by far the most common type of Hodgkin lymphoma in the United States. It characteristically presents in the neck and/or mediastinum of young females.

Lymphocyte depletion Hodgkin lymphoma may present in adults or elderly patients as a febrile illness with pancytopenia or lymphocytopenia, hepatomegaly, abnormal liver function tests, and no peripheral lymphadenopathy, or it may manifest the usual clinical presentation of Hodgkin lymphoma. This form is extremely rare in children, in whom nodular sclerosis and lymphocyte predominance predominate greatly.

Mediastinal involvement is the rule in nodular sclerosis, in constant in mixed cellularity and lymphocyte depletion, and exceptional in NLPHL. The risk of abdominal involvement is greater in patients with B symptoms and in lymphocyte depletion or mixed cellularity types; the lowest risk is for asymptomatic females with nodular sclerosis histology (6%).

The diagnosis of Hodgkin lymphoma should be questioned for any lymphoma involving Waldeyer's ring, the skin, and the gastrointestinal tract, especially if this happens to be the first manifestation of the disease. Most of these cases are examples of non-Hodgkin lymphomas with Reed-Sternberg-like cells.

Patients with Hodgkin lymphoma often have defects in cellular immunity, which leads to an increased susceptibility to some infections. However, a diagnosis of Hodgkin lymphoma should be viewed with suspicion if it presents as a complication of a natural immune deficiency, immunosuppression, or other immune diseases. Although indubitable cases of this association exist (particularly in patients with ataxia–telangiectasia and with HIV infection), most of these cases actually represent large cell sarcomas containing binucleated immunoblasts morphologically similar to Reed-Sternberg cells. HIV-associated Hodgkin lymphoma tends to present at a high stage and to run an aggressive clinical course.

Spread

Most cases of Hodgkin lymphoma begin in lymph nodes and spread from there to other lymph node groups and to extranodal sites. Important information has been acquired in regard to the frequency and significance of this spread as a result of an aggressive diagnostic approach, particularly with the use of laparotomy as a routine staging procedure.

1. *Direct extension*: The disease may spread to the perinodal tissues, sometimes extensively, and result in a fusion of the involved nodes. In advanced cases, direct invasion of skin, skeletal muscle, and other sites can occur. Mediastinal Hodgkin lymphoma can extend by continuity into the large vessels, lung, and chest wall.

2. *Other lymph node groups*: Most cases of Hodgkin lymphoma spread by involvement of adjacent lymph node groups. This contiguous manner of spread is particularly common in the nodular sclerosis and lymphocyte predominance types. Nodal spread has been evaluated with lymphangiogram, CT scan, and staging laparotomy. When it was carried out with some frequency, lymphangiography had an overall diagnostic accuracy in excess of 90%; it was more effective in detecting involvement below the level of the second lumbar vertebra but inconsistent for nodes situated higher in the periaortic area. Approximately 30% of patients with negative lympha-ngiograms in whom the para-aortic nodes were left untreated later demonstrated disease below the diaphragm. Of the nodes biopsied at laparotomy during the course of a staging procedure, the most likely to be involved were those located in the splenic hilum and retroperitoneum. Mesenteric nodes are almost always spared.

3. *Spleen*: A spleen weighing 400 g or more is practically always histologically positive. The converse is not true: Spleens below this weight are involved in a high proportion of cases. The focal nature of the disease calls for a careful gross examination of this organ. The specimens should be sectioned throughout in thin slices, and every suspicious area should be examined

microscopically. If no nodules are detected on gross inspection, the chances of finding Hodgkin lymphoma in random microscopic sections are negligible. Splenic involvement is thought to represent a critical stage in the spread of Hodgkin lymphoma and is an early manifestation of blood vessel dissemination. The approximate number of tumor nodules present in the spleen should be indicated because of their relation to prognosis; specifically, it should be stated whether there are five or more. It is not important to subclassify the disease in the spleen into the specific type.

4. *Liver*: Hepatic disease is almost invariably associated with splenic and retroperitoneal lymph node involvement and with so-called 'B symptoms'. Clinical assessment of liver involvement is quite unreliable. Care should be exercised in distinguishing involvement by Hodgkin lymphoma from benign lymphoid aggregates, some of which may show mild atypia.

5. *Bone marrow*

6. *Others*: Practically any other organ can show secondary involvement by Hodgkin lymphoma, such as the lung, skin, gastrointestinal tract, and central nervous system.

Staging

The current staging classification for Hodgkin lymphoma was established by the Ann Arbor Workshop in 1971 and modified at Cotswolds in 1989 (Box 2). Clinical staging refers to all procedures short of laparotomy. It includes physical examination, bone marrow aspiration and biopsy, clinical laboratory evaluation, and numerous radiographic studies. Chest X-ray and thoracic and abdominal CT studies have become the norm, and these are supplemented in some centers by bipedal lymphangiogram and gallium scans. Pathologic staging used to refer to the findings at staging laparotomy during which liver, splenectomy, and biopsies of retroperitoneal lymph nodes, liver, and bone marrow were performed. Although much important information has been obtained from the performance of routine staging laparotomy in patients with Hodgkin lymphoma, the procedure is now used only sparingly, the reasons being the increased diagnostic power of radiographic techniques, the high efficiency of current therapies, and the occurrence of postsurgical complications, particularly in the pediatric population.

Box 2: Ann Arbor staging classification for Hodgkin lymphoma (as modified at Costwolds)

Stage I

Involvement of a single lymph node region (I) or a single extralymphatic organ or site (Ig)

Stage II

Involvement of two or more lymph node regions on the same side of the diaphragm (II) or localized involvement of an extralymphatic organ or site (IIg)

Stage III

Involvement of lymph node regions on both sides of the diaphragm (III) or localized involvement of an extralymphatic organ or site (IIIg) or spleen (IIIg) or both (IIIse)

Stage IV

Diffuse or disseminated involvement of one or more extralymphatic organs with or without associated lymph node involvement. The organ(s) involved should be identified by a symbol[a]

From Warnke RA, Weiss LM, Chan JKC, Cleary ML, Dorfman RF. Tumors of the lymph nodes and spleen. Atlas of tumor pathology, series 3, fascicle 14. Washington, DC, 1995, Armed Forces Institute of Pathology.

[a] *A, Asymptomatic; B, fever >38°C previous month, sweats previous month, weight loss >10% of body weight previous 6 months; X, bulk (>10 cm for lymph node, >1/3 of internal transverse diameter of thorax at >5/6 on a posteroanterior chest radiograph).*

Treatment

The treatment of patients with early-stage Hodgkin lymphoma is one of the success stories of modern oncology. The two pillars of therapy are radiation therapy and chemotherapy, the choice being largely dependent on the stage of the disease and the bias of the individual centers. Increasingly, chemotherapy is adopted as the mainstay of treatment. Bone marrow transplantation is used in selected cases.

Prognosis

The current overall 5-year survival rate of Hodgkin lymphoma is over 75%.

Non-Hodgkin Lymphoma

The classification of non-Hodgkin lymphoma that was most widely used until the early 1980s in the United States and many other countries was that proposed by Rappaport in 1966 (Table 7.9). This represented a slight modification of the classification that Gall and Rappaport had presented at a seminar of the American Society of Clinical Pathologists held in New Orleans, Louisiana, in 1963. This, in turn, was based on the classification proposed by Gall and Mallory as part of their comprehensive critical study of 618 lymphomas. Rappaport's classification was, of necessity, based entirely on morphologic grounds. Numerous independent clinicopathologic studies have shown its reproducibility, usefulness, and clinical relevance. However, application of the remarkable advances in the fields of immunology, cytogenetics, and molecular pathology in the past 40 years to the study of lymphomas has shown that these can be viewed as clonal expansions of the normal anatomic and functional components of the immune system. Most of them have been studied using immunologic and molecular genetic markers and, as a result, have been 'typed' as to their normal counterparts, from which presumably they arose. This 'functional' approach, championed by Lukesin in the United States and by Lennert in Germany, incorporated a number of entities and showed that a functional classification of lymphoma was possible to some extent on the basis of morphologic interpretation of routinely stained sections (Table 7.9). Independent of this, aggressive clinical investigations coupled with staging laparotomies provided a wealth of new information on the sites of predilection and spread of the lymphomas according to type. The results obtained with these investigations pointed to some inaccuracies and other deficiencies of Rappaport's classification and the need to revise it, taking into account all these new data.

Five new classifications were proposed, which, needless to say, resulted in a confusing state of affairs for both pathologists and clinicians.

Because there was no clear cut evidence that one classification was significantly superior to the others, the National Cancer Institute sponsored a retrospective study of 1175 cases of non-Hodgkin lymphoma, which were classified according to the different categories by the investigators who proposed them, as well as by a panel of 'control' pathologists. Analysis of the data showed that all six classifications were successful in predicting the prognosis in a large number of lymphoma patients and that no classification appeared clearly superior to any other in this respect. It also confirmed that lymphomas with a follicular pattern

Table 7.9: Major historic classification schemes of non-Hodgkin lymphoma

Rappaport	*Lukes and Collins*	*Kiel*
Nodular	Undefined cell type	Low-grade malignancy
Lymphocytic, well differentiated	T cell type	Lymphocytic
	Small lymphocytic	Chronic lymphocytic leukemia
Lymphocytic, poorly differentiated	Sézary-mycosis fungoides (cerebriform)	Other
Mixed (lymphocytic and histiocytic)	Convoluted lymphocytic	Lymphoplasmacytoid
Histiocytic		Centrocytic
Diffuse	Immunoblastic sarcoma (T cell)	Centroblastic-centrocytic
Lymphocytic, well differentiated	Small lymphocytic	Follicular, without sclerosis
Without plasmacytoid features	B cell type	Follicular, with sclerosis
	Small lymphocytic	
With plasmacytoid features	Plasmacytoid lymphocytic	Follicular and diffuse, without sclerosis
Lymphocytic, poorly differentiated	Follicular center cell[a]	Follicular and diffuse, with sclerosis
Without plasmacytoid features	Small cleaved	
	Large cleaved	Diffuse
With plasmacytoid features	Small noncleaved	Unclassified
Lymphoblastic	Large noncleaved	High-grade malignancy
Convoluted	Immunoblastic sarcoma (B cell)	Centroblastic
Nonconvoluted	Histiocytic	Lymphoblastic
Mixed (lymphocytic and histiocytic)	Unclassified	Burkitt type
	Composite	Convoluted cell type
Histiocytic		Other (unclassified)
Without sclerosis		Immunoblastic
With sclerosis		Unclassified
Burkitt tumor		Unclassified
Undifferentiated		Composite
Unclassified		
Composite		

Contd.

Contd.

International formulation

Low grade	Intermediate grade	High grade	Miscellaneous
ML,[b] small lymphocytic	ML, follicular, predominantly large cell	ML, large cell, immunoblastic	Composite
Consistent with chronic lymphocytic leukemia	With diffuse areas	Plasmacytoid	Mycosis fungoides
		Clear cell	Histiocytic
	With sclerosis	Polymorphous	Extramedullary plasmacytoma
Plasmacytoid	ML, diffuse, small cleaved cell	With epithelioid cell component	Unclassifiable
ML, follicular, predominantly small cleaved cell	With sclerosis	ML, lymphoblastic	Other
	ML, diffuse, mixed (small and large cell)	Convoluted	
With diffuse areas		Nonconvoluted	
With sclerosis	With sclerosis	ML, small noncleaved cell	
ML, follicular, mixed (small cleaved and large cell)	With epithelioid cell component	Burkitt	
	ML, diffuse, large cell	With follicular areas	
With diffuse areas	Cleaved cell		
With sclerosis	Noncleaved cell		
	With sclerosis		

[a] Subdivided into: (1) follicular, follicular and diffuse, and diffuse; and (2) without sclerosis and with sclerosis.

[b] Malignant lymphoma.

of growth (a feature consistently identified by all reviewers) had a more favorable prognosis than those with diffuse patterns within the same cytologic subtypes. This was true whether the nodularity was extensive or only partial. Finally, it confirmed the suspicion that within the 'histiocytic lymphoma' category of Rappaport, there was a variety of morphologically recognizable neoplasms with a different natural history. As a result of the analysis of these 1175 cases, the investigators involved in this study proposed a new classification (hiding it under the euphemism 'Working Formulation') of non-Hodgkin malignant lymphomas, based primarily on light microscopic differences as seen in sections stained with hematoxylin–eosin, that showed a good correlation with survival. Ten major types plus a miscellaneous group were identified, and these were subdivided into three major prognostic groups that were of favorable, intermediate, and unfavorable prognosis, respectively.

Although this de facto classification gained some degree of acceptability, it was viewed by many as a compromise rather than a conceptual advance, just as the Rye classification of Hodgkin lymphoma had been seen as a compromise (not necessarily for the better) over the Lukes-Butler classification. It was also pointed out from the very beginning that the Working Formulation did not take into account all the entities that had been recognized at that time. This, plus the continuing advances that have been made in the field, has led to additions and other substantial changes to the scheme.

In the mid 1990s, an international group of hematopathologists prepared a list of lymphoid neoplasms that they felt could be recognized with available techniques and which appeared to be clinically distinctive. The approach was strictly pragmatic, in the sense that the list included only those categories that appeared reasonably identifiable as such, without attempting to always relate them to normal stages of lymphoid differentiation. This attempt, to which the cute term REAL (Revised European American Lymphoma Classification) was given, has been the model upon which the new WHO classification of tumors of hematopoietic and lymphoid tissues published in 2001 and updated in 2008 is based (Box 3).

Box 3: REAL/WHO 2001/WHO 2008 classification

B cell neoplasms

Precursor B cell neoplasm

    B lymphoblastic leukemia/lymphoma

Mature B cell neoplasms

    Chronic lymphocytic leukemia/small lymphocytic lymphoma

    B cell prolymphocytic leukemia

    Lymphoplasmacytic lymphoma

    Splenic marginal zone lymphoma

    Hairy cell leukemia

    Plasma cell neoplasms (plasma cell myeloma/plasmacytoma)

    Extranodal marginal zone lymphoma of mucosa-associated lymphoid tissue (MALT-lymphoma)

    Nodal marginal zone lymphoma

    Follicular lymphoma

Primary cutaneous follicle center lymphoma

Mantle cell lymphoma

Diffuse large B cell lymphomas (DLBCL)

DLBCL, not otherwise specified

T cell/histiocyte-rich large B cell lymphoma

Primary DLBCL of the central nervous system

Primary cutaneous DLBCL, leg-type

Epstein-Barr virus + DLBCL of the elderly

Primary mediastinal (thymic) large B cell lymphoma

Intravascular large B cell lymphoma

DLBCL associated with chronic inflammation

Lymphomatoidgranulomatosis

ALK+ large B cell lymphoma

Plasmablastic lymphoma

Large B cell lymphoma arising in HHV8-associated multicentric Castleman disease

Primary effusion lymphoma

Burkitt lymphoma

B cell lymphoma, unclassifiable, with features intermediate between diffuse large B cell lymphoma and Burkitt lymphoma

B cell lymphoma, unclassifiable, with features intermediate between diffuse large B cell lymphoma and classical Hodgkin lymphoma

T cell and NK cell neoplasms

Precursor T cell neoplasms

T lymphoblastic leukemia/lymphoma

Mature T cell and NK cell neoplasms

T cell prolymphocytic leukemia

T cell large granular lymphocytic leukemia

Aggressive NK cell leukemia

Adult T cell leukemia/lymphoma

Epstein-Barr virus + T cell lymphoproliferative diseases of childhood

Extranodal NK/T cell lymphoma, nasal type

Enteropathy-associated T cell lymphoma

Hepatosplenic T cell lymphoma

Subcutaneous panniculitis-like T cell lymphoma

Mycosis fungoides

Sézary syndrome

Primary cutaneous CD30+ T cell lymphoproliferative disorders

Primary cutaneous peripheral T cell lymphomas, rare subtypes

Peripheral T cell lymphoma, not otherwise specified
Angioimmunoblastic T cell lymphoma
Anaplastic large cell lymphoma, ALK+
Anaplastic large cell lymphoma, ALK–

Small Lymphocytic Lymphoma

Small lymphocytic lymphoma (commonly referred to as 'chronic lymphocytic leukemia/small lymphocytic lymphoma') preferentially occurs in middle-aged and elderly individuals. The patients often have a few or no symptoms, the evolution is prolonged, and the survival is very good. It is not unusual to find the disease incidentally in lymph node dissections done for carcinoma of one type or another.

The architecture of the node in small lymphocytic lymphoma is massively and monotonously effaced by a population of small round lymphocytes with clumped chromatin, inconspicuous nucleoli, barely visible cytoplasm, and scanty mitotic activity. There are also variable numbers of larger cells (prolymphocytes and paraimmunoblasts) with vesicular nuclei and distinct nucleoli, singly or in small aggregates that simulate germinal centers. These formations (known as proliferative centers, growth centers, or pseudofollicles) have an increased number of Ki-67-positive cells. This feature, which is apparently of no prognostic significance, should not lead to confusion with follicular lymphoma or NLPHL. As a matter of fact, the presence of these pseudofollicular formations and of prolymphocytes/paraimmunoblasts corroborates the diagnosis of small lymphocytic lymphoma as opposed to mantle cell lymphoma.

The distribution of the disease is usually diffuse, but on occasions it is confined to the marginal zone, the perifollicular regions, or the interfollicular regions surrounding benign lymphoid follicles, the latter pattern being referred to as *interfollicular small lymphocytic lymphoma*. Some cases show a propensity for invasion of the wall of veins. Extranodal extension is seen in approximately one-third of the cases.

Cases of small lymphocytic lymphomas can be divided into three categories: (1) those with absolute lymphocytosis (i.e. chronic lymphocytic leukemia); (2) those associated with monoclonal gammopathy (50% of which have bone marrow involvement); and (3) those with neither; the latter are often accompanied by hypogammaglobulinemia. There are no statistical differences in survival between these three groups and no appreciable morphologic differences between the first and the third groups. In the cases associated with monoclonal gammopathy, some or most of the neoplastic lymphocytes may exhibit morphologic signs of plasmacytoid differentiation (as evidenced by oval shape, lateralization of the nucleus, appearance of a perinuclear halo, and pyroninophilia) and admixture of plasma cells. Effacement of the nodal architecture is generally not as complete as with the usual type. These cases are referred to as *small lymphocytic lymphoma with plasmacytic differentiation* and are discussed further in the section on lymphoma and dysproteinemia.

Immunohistochemically, small lymphocytic lymphomas are always of B cell type. Monoclonal immunoglobulins, including both IgM and IgD types, are consistently found on their surface. They differ from the B lymphocytes of follicular lymphoma in the intensity and appearance of the reaction (brighter and more clumped in the latter), as well as by their lesser content of complement receptors. They are usually CD20+ (not uncommonly weak), CD5+, CD23+, CD43+, and cyclin D1. At the molecular level, Ig heavy and light chain genes are rearranged. Cyto-genetically, trisomy 12 has been reported in one-third of the cases (said to be associated with a poor prognosis), and abnormalities of 13q in up to one-fourth (said to be associated with a good survival). Cases showing somatic hypermutation of the immuno-globulin gene (with negative staining for ZAP-70 being a surrogate marker) are associated with a favorable prognosis.

There is a rare small lymphoid cell neoplasm of T lineage which is clinically and pathologically different from small lymphocytic lymphoma, and which therefore should not be classified within this category. The cells are usually somewhat larger, have numerous azurophilic granules, and contain large amounts of acid phosphatase and β-glucuronidase.

Follicular Lymphoma

Follicular (nodular) lymphoma is a B cell neoplasm that recapi-tulates the architectural and cytologic features of the normal secondary lymphoid follicle. This tumor comprises up to 40% of all adult non-Hodgkin lymphomas in the United States, but in other countries the relative incidence is much lower. Most cases occur in elderly individuals. It is very unusual under 20 years of age and relatively uncommon in blacks. Most of the cases diagnosed in the past as follicular lymphomas in children actually represent NLPHL or reactive follicular hyperplasia. However, well-documented cases of follicular lymphoma in children are on record.

Grossly and at low-power examination, the most distinctive feature of these tumors is the nodular pattern of growth. Rappaport et al., have carefully outlined in a classic article the differential points between these neoplastic nodules and the reactive follicles of follicular hyperplasia. With progression of the disease, this distinct nodularity becomes blurred, and eventually most of the proliferation acquires a diffuse pattern. The cytologic composition of the neoplastic nodules is characterized by a mixture in different proportions of small and large lymphoid cells, both of which resemble their normal follicular counterparts. The small cells have scanty cytoplasm and an irregular, elongated cleaved nucleus with prominent indentations and infoldings; the size is similar to or slightly larger than that of normal lymphocytes, the chromatin is coarse, and the nucleolus is inconspicuous. These cells have been variously referred to as germinocytes, centrocytes, poorly differentiated lymphocytes, and small cleaved follicular center cells. The large cells are two or three times the size of normal lymphocytes; they have a distinct rim of cytoplasm and a vesicular nucleus with one or three nucleoli often adjacent to the nuclear membrane. These cells, which have a rapid turnover rate and probably represent the proliferating component of the tumor, have been designated over the years as germinoblasts, centroblasts, histiocytes, large (cleaved or noncleaved) follicular center cells, large lymphoid cells, and lymphoblasts. Some may be binucleated and simulate Reed-Sternberg cells. It ought to be mentioned here that another type of large cell seen in follicular lymphoma is the non-neoplastic follicular dendritic cell, for the very reason that the tumor involves lymphoid follicles; it is recognized because of its finely dispersed chromatin, the lack of identifiable cell boundaries, and the inconspicuousness of the nucleolus. In contrast to their counterparts in benign follicles, these cells show a little or no immunoreactivity for fascin.

Immunohistochemically, the follicles of follicular lymphoma (including all its variants) are composed of a monoclonal population of B cells admixed with variable numbers of non-neoplastic small T cells, macrophages, and follicular dendritic cells, corresponding to the cellular composition of a normal germinal center. The tumor cells express pan-B antigens, such as CD19, CD20, CD22, and CD79a, in addition to HLA-DR. They also express surface and/or cytoplasmic immunoglobulins (usually of the IgM type) with light chain restriction. CD10 (CALLA), a germinal center cell marker, is detected in approximately 60–70% of the cases. This marker can aid in distinction from reactive follicular hyperplasia when significant numbers of CD10+ cells are found in the interfollicular zone as an indication of interfollicular invasion. BCL6, another germinal center cell marker, is expressed in most cases. CD5 and CD43 are usually negative.

The BCL2 protein can be identified immunohistochemically in approximately 85% of cases, and is thus one of the most useful markers for the differential diagnosis with reactive follicular hyperplasia (BCL2 negative), although it is important to realize that BCL2 negativity does not totally rule out follicular lymphoma. Immunostaining for BCL2 cannot be used for distinction of follicular lymphoma from other low-grade B cell lymphomas, because the latter are commonly BCL2 positive; to deal with such a diagnostic problem, immunostaining for follicular center cell markers such as CD10 and BCL6 is more helpful.

Follicular lymphoma shows clonal rearrangements of the immunoglobulin genes, which also feature hypermutations and ongoing somatic mutations, as characteristic of follicle center B cells.

The hallmark genetic alteration of follicular lymphoma is t(14;18)(q32;q21), found in 85% of cases. The chromosomal translocation juxtaposes IGH with the BCL2 gene, driving overexpression of BCL2 protein, an anti-apoptotic molecule located in the inner mitochondrial membrane whose expression is typically switched off in normal follicle center B cells. As a result of aberrant BCL2 expression, the neoplastic follicle center cells do not undergo apoptosis. Thus follicular lymphoma results more from cell accumulation than cell proliferation. Although BCL2 rearrangement is also seen in some cases of diffuse large B cell lymphoma, demonstration of this molecular alteration provides a good support for a diagnosis of follicular lymphoma in the appropriate context, such as distinction from atypical follicular hyperplasia, marginal zone lymphoma with follicular growth pattern and mantle cell lymphoma. For this purpose, FISH is more sensitive than PCR. Certain types of follicular lymphoma uncommonly or do not exhibit BCL2 rearrangement, including pediatric follicular lymphoma, primary cutaneous follicle center lymphoma, and grade 3b follicular lymphoma.

Depending on the relative proportion of small and large cells, follicular lymphomas are subdivided into three categories, respectively designated in the WHO classification as follows:

1. Grade 1, with 0–15 centroblasts (large nucleolated cells) per high-power field.
2. Grade 2, with 6–15 centroblasts per high-power field.
3. Grade 3, with more than 15 centroblasts per high-power field. Cases with admixed centrocytes are referred to as grade 3a, while cases with solid sheets of centroblasts are referred to as grade 3b. In the first category, which is the most common, mitotic activity is infrequent. Conversely, the appearance of large cells is often accompanied by a parallel increase in the number of mitoses.

Mantle Cell Lymphoma

Mantle cell lymphoma is a low-grade neoplasm also known as intermediate lymphocytic, mantle zone, centrocytic, and diffuse small cleaved cell lymphoma. It comprises from 3% to 10% of all cases of non-Hodgkin lymphoma. Like follicular lymphoma, it usually occurs in middle-aged and elderly individuals. The low-power appearance is largely that of a diffuse lymphoma, although there may be a suggestion of nodularity accentuated by the occasional presence of small germinal center-like structures ('naked' germinal centers). The neoplastic cells are small, and often show irregular and indented nuclear contours similar to those seen in small cleaved cell follicular lymphoma. On occasion, some of the tumor cells show plasma cell differentiation. In some cases, the tumor cells have larger nuclei with more dispersed chromatin and a higher proliferative fraction ('blastoid' or 'pleomorphic' variant). Sometimes one form is seen evolving into the other, an event confirmed by clonality studies. The blastoid form of mantle cell lymphoma (and sometimes also the classic form) may be accompanied by blood, bone marrow, and spleen involvement ('mantle cell leukemia').

Two common morphologic features of mantle cell lymphoma are hyalinized blood vessels and a scattering of epithelioid histiocytes, the former representing an important diagnostic clue and the latter sometimes resulting in a starry sky appearance.

The immunocytochemical profile suggests that mantle cell lymphoma is a distinct type of malignant lymphoma having the features of the lymphocytes of primary follicles and / or the mantle zones of secondary follicles, i.e. naive pregerminal center cells. The tumor cells are positive for immunoglobulins (IgM and often also IgD), B cell-associated antigens, and CD5. The general absence of CD23 is useful in distinguishing mantle cell lymphoma from small lymphocytic lymphoma, and the presence of CD5 is useful in the differential diagnosis with follicular and marginal zone lymphomas. It should be remarked, however, that CD5 expression is not always present in mantle cell lymphoma and can be present in some diffuse large B cell lymphomas apparently unrelated to mantle cell lymphoma. As explained below, overexpression of cyclin D1 protein is a constant and nearly specific feature of mantle cell lymphoma, which therefore becomes of great importance in its differential diagnosis. Although immunohistochemical demonstration of cyclin D1 has been difficult in the past, this has now become easy with the availability of a rabbit monoclonal antibody against cyclin D1.

Marginal Zone B cell Lymphoma

Marginal zone B cell lymphoma is the generic term used in the REAL/WHO schemes to designate an increasingly larger family of low-grade B cell lymphomas comprised of a heterogeneous population of small B cells. The concept represents a grouping of entities that had been described separately, most of them at extranodal sites. There appears to be considerable clinical, morphologic, and immunohistochemical overlap among the three entities (extranodal, nodal, and splenic). Consequently, the proposal has been made that they represent a related family of neoplasms showing morphologic evidence of differentiation into cells of marginal zone type. These cells are thought to have the capacity to mature into both monocytoid B cells and plasma cells, and to display tissue-specific homing patterns. A corollary of this proposal is that the various clinical syndromes may be the result of the homing pattern of the specific neoplastic clone. The proposal has been generally accepted, although it has been pointed out that important clinical and molecular genetic differences among the subgroups and even within a given subgroup exist.

1. *Nodal marginal zone lymphoma (monocytoid B cell lymphoma)*: This term has been used for a tumor of small to medium-sized

lymphocytes with round or slightly indented nuclei and relatively abundant clear cytoplasm, usually located in lymph nodes, hence its alternate designation as nodal. The tumor cells have been regarded as the neoplastic counterpart of the monocytoid B lymphocytes found in lymph node sinuses in toxoplasmosis and other reactive disorders. Plasmacytoid features are prominent in some cases. The pattern of involvement is predominantly sinusal and interfollicular, but cases have been seen with 'follicular colonization' and with 'floral' features. Clinically, the disease is more common in women, and can be localized or generalized at presentation. Some patients have suffered from autoimmune disorders such as Sjögren disease. In all cases, the possibility of nodal spread from an extranodal marginal zone lymphoma has to be excluded by clinical workup. Histologic transformation to large cell lymphoma has been documented in some cases.

Diffuse Mixed (small and large cell) Lymphoma

Diffuse mixed lymphoma is not a specific lymphoma type but a heterogeneous category composed of lymphomas of various types that share a mixed composition of large and small lymphoid cells. It includes: (1) the diffuse mixed cell form of follicular lymphoma; (2) peripheral T cell lymphoma; (3) lymphoplasmacytic lymphoma with an increased number of immunoblasts (also known as polymorphic immunocytoma); (4) T cell-rich large B cell lymphoma; and (5) some examples of marginal zone B cell lymphoma with an admixture of large cells; and probably others. The differential diagnosis among these various entities is based on a combination of clinical, morphologic, and immunohisto-chemical criteria.

Diffuse Large B cell Lymphoma

Diffuse large B cell lymphoma (DLBCL) is the most complex and heterogeneous of all the non-Hodgkin lymphomas. The term replaces the old histiocytic lymphoma, which in turn replaced the older reticulum cell sarcoma. It is characterized morphologically by large size of the cells, vesicular nuclei with prominent nucleoli, and relatively abundant cytoplasm, and immunophenotypically by expression of B-lineage markers.

Plasmablastic lymphoma: Plasmablastic lymphoma is a B cell neoplasm that corresponds to the differentiation stage between a B immunoblast and a plasma cell. It is an incompletely characterized entity without universal agreement on the minimum diagnostic criteria. Notwithstanding, this is an important type of DLBCL to recognize because it poses significant diagnostic problems (the diagnosis can be difficult because conventional lymphoid markers are not uncommonly all negative) and has therapeutic implications (probably not responsive to rituximab due to lack of CD20 expression). Plasmablastic lymphoma is highly aggressive. It can affect HIV-infected subjects (most commonly oral cavity) or immunocompetent subjects, either involving lymph node or extranodal sites. Conceptually, there are several subgroups with similar morphology and immunophenotype: (1) ALK+ large B cell lymphoma; (2) primary effusion lymphoma; and (3) plasmablastic lymphoma, not otherwise specified. However, by convention the first two subgroups are not labeled as plasmablastic lymphoma. Morphologically, plasmablastic lymphoma comprises large cells with vesicular nuclei, single centrally located prominent nucleolus or multiple peripheral nucleoli, abundant basophilic cytoplasm, and paranuclear hof. The neoplastic population is monomorphic or shows admixed immature plasma cells. The immunophenotype mirrors that of normal plasma cells, being CD45–, CD20–, CD79a+/–, PAX5–, CD38+, VS38c+, CD138+, MUM1+. There is variable expression of cytoplasmic immunoglobulin. EBV is positive in 60–75% of cases, and HHV8 is positive in a small proportion of cases. In practice, it is extremely difficult to distinguish plasmablastic lymphoma from anaplastic/plasmablastic plasmacytoma.

ALK+ large B cell lymphoma: This is an uncommon form of DLBCL with plasmablastic differentiation and a poor prognosis. The tumor cells have an immunoblastic or plasmablastic appearance, and sinusoidal infiltration is common. Since they can appear deceptively cohesive, they are not uncommonly misinterpreted as carcinoma cells. The immunophenotype is characteristic of plasmablastic lymphoma, CD30 is negative, and IgA is commonly positive. The commonest molecular alteration is t(2; 17) (p23; q23), which fuses the ALK gene with the CLTC gene. Since CLTC encodes a granule-associated protein, immunostaining for ALK is typically in the form of cytoplasmic granules. Rare cases exhibit t(2;5) with NPM–ALK fusion as in ALK+ ALCL, and ALK immunoreactivity is similarly nuclear-cytoplasmic. EBV and HHV8 are negative.

Primary effusion lymphoma. This is a DLBCL with plasmablastic differentiation, occurring predominantly in patients with AIDS, and showing a strong association with HHV8 and EBV. A solid tissue counterpart also exists.

Peripheral (post-thymic) T cell and NK-cell Lymphomas

Peripheral (post-thymic) T cell and NK cell lymphoma is the generic group given to a family of tumors composed of neoplastic lymphocytes with phenotypic and genotypic features of mature T cells or NK cells. This is an extremely heterogeneous group of lesions, many of them occurring primarily at extranodal sites, and which have received a myriad of designations. Most of them were identified as entities long before their peripheral T cell or NK cell nature was ascertained. They include:

- *Mycosis fungoides* and *Sézary syndrome*
- *NK/T cell lymphoma, nasal type*, which includes most of the cases traditionally diagnosed as lethal midline granuloma
- *Enteropathy-associated T cell lymphoma*, which includes most of the cases of intestinal lymphoma arising as a complication of celiac disease
- *Hepatosplenic T cell lymphoma*
- *Subcutaneous panniculitis-like T cell lymphoma*
- *Angioimmunoblastic T cell lymphoma*
- The tumor type originally described by Lennert as malignant lymphoma with a constantly high number of epithelioid cells and variously known as *Lennert lymphoma* and *lymphoepithelioid lymphoma*
- *Adult T cell leukemia/lymphoma*, an HTLV-1-related pleomorphic T cell lymphoma occurring in an endemic form in Japan.
- Miscellaneous peripheral T cell lymphomas described under the designations of T cell immunoblastic sarcoma, T cell lymphoma with multilobated nuclei, erythrophagocytic T cell lymphoma, T zone lymphoma, peripheral T cell lymphoma with perifollicular growth pattern, and nodal CD8+ cytotoxic T cell lymphoma.
- *Anaplastic large cell lymphoma* and its variants

Anaplastic Large Cell Lymphoma

Anaplastic large cell lymphoma (ALCL, also known as Ki-1 lymphoma) is characterized by highly atypical and pleomorphic neoplastic cells with expression of the activation marker CD30. Although previously a secondary form supervening on other types of lymphoma (such as mycosis fungoides and Hodgkin lymphoma) was recognized in addition to the more common *de novo* (primary) form, currently only the latter is acceptable for the category of ALCL according to the WHO classification. There is also a change from the initial characterization of this entity, in that only cases of T or null-cell lineage are included in the category of ALCL; cases of B-lineage are simply diagnosed as 'diffuse large B cell lymphoma, anaplastic variant'.

Burkitt Lymphoma

Burkitt lymphoma is a high-grade malignant lymphoma composed of germinal center B cells which can present in three clinical settings:

1. *Endemic*: This occurs in the equatorial strip of Africa and is the most common form of childhood malignancy in this area. The patients characteristically present with jaw and orbital lesions. Involvement of the gastrointestinal tract, ovaries, kidney, and breast are also common.

2. *Sporadic*: This is seen throughout the world. It affects mainly children and adolescents, and has a greater tendency for involvement of the abdominal cavity than the endemic form.

3. *Immunodeficiency-associated*: This is seen primarily in association with HIV infection and often occurs as the initial manifestation of the disease.

In all three forms peripheral lymphadenopathy is rare and, when present, usually limited to a single group. Bone marrow involvement is common in the late stage of the disease, but leukemic manifestations are very rare.

Microscopically, the pattern of growth of Burkitt lymphoma is usually diffuse, although early cases may show preferential involvement of germinal centers. The tumor cells are medium sized (10–25 μm) and round. The nuclei are round or oval and have *several* prominent basophilic nucleoli. The chromatin is coarse and the nuclear membrane is rather thick. The cytoplasm is easily identifiable; it is amphophilic in hematoxylin–eosin-stained preparations and strongly pyroninophilic. Fat-containing small vacuoles are present; these are particularly well appreciated in touch preparations. Mitoses are numerous, and a prominent starry sky pattern is the rule, although by no means pathognomonic. There are also many admixed apoptotic bodies. In well-fixed material, the cytoplasm of individual cells 'squares off', forming acute angles in which the membranes of adjacent cells abut on each other. Occasionally, the tumor is accompanied by a florid granulomatous reaction. Ultrastructurally, the main features are abundant ribosomes, frequent lipid inclusions, lack of glycogen particles, and presence of nuclear pockets or projections.

Two morphologic variants of Burkitt lymphoma are recognized. In the form with *plasmacytoid differentiation*, which is more common in HIV-related cases, some tumor cells exhibit eccentric basophilic cytoplasm containing immunoglobulin and a single central nucleolus. In the *atypical* or *pleomorphic* form, the cell size is larger and a distinct pleomorphism is evident. Most of the cells have a well-defined rim of cytoplasm; their nucleus contains a large, eosinophilic nucleolus. Binucleated and multinucleated cells are common. Phagocytosis of nuclear debris by reactive histiocytes is as common as in the classic form, resulting in a starry sky appearance. The pattern of growth is generally diffuse, but areas of minimal nodularity may be encountered. Clinically, gastrointestinal involvement is less common and bone marrow involvement more frequent than in the classic form. The clinical course is said to be more aggressive although the response to therapy is similar. In the 2008 WHO classification, it is recommended that the term 'atypical Burkitt lymphoma' be dropped; a case would be simply classified as 'Burkitt lymphoma' if the immunophenotypic and genotypic features are compatible.

Burkitt lymphomas are of B cell lineage. They express immunoglobulins (predominantly IgM), invariably associated with heavy and light chain restriction. B cell-specific antigens (such as CD19, CD20, and CD22) and B cell-associated antigens (such as CD24 and HLA-DR) are present. Most cases also express the germinal center cell markers CD10 and BCL6. They are negative for the activation markers CD25 and CD30. In contrast to lymphoblastic lymphoma, they do not express TdT. The most helpful immunohistochemical profile to aid in diagnosis of Burkitt lymphoma includes CD20+, CD10+, BCL2– (although weak staining can be seen in some cases), and a Ki-67 index over 95%.

Index